Testimonials

"Thank you for the respectful, sensitive way that you work with people. Body image, colors, clothing, and vanity always confused me. Raised in a conservative home in a rural area, dressing mostly meant: be clean, groomed and pressed when possible. In different home and work cultures, I realize our image gets projected one way or another. You are an answer to solve the fashion confusion, consumerism and clothing care and storage. I've learned clothes can be a fun hobby adding fulfillment to life. It makes getting up in the morning brighter. Jill, people and clothing are your palette. What an artist!"
Joy Kliber – L.I.C.S.W. Management Consultant

"I can't thank Jill enough! I'm telling you, I've received so many compliments. Especially from my husband, he has gone out of his way to express his approval for my new look."
June Chapko – Author and Networking Leader

"Simply Beautiful is MORE than another makeup manual. It's a refreshing journey for women, leading them to both inner and outer beauty. Jill shows how the simple use of color, make-up, style, and organization improve every woman's life. Then she feeds our soul with ageless wisdom. The result: Simply beautiful ways to be simply beautiful."
Joy E. DeKok – Christian Author and Speaker

"As I train speakers and encourage them to improve their stage presence and develop their personal persona, I regularly recommend Jill's services. Her approach combines color, style, and practicality. Jill's presentations have been a hit at every conference at which I have invited her to share her expertise. It is from this background that I refer women to get Jill's book."
Marita Littauer – President, CLASServices Inc.

SIMPLY BEAUTIFUL

Inside and Out

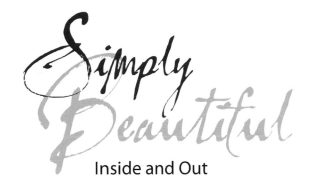

Simply Beautiful
Inside and Out

By Jill Krieger Swanson

River City Press, Inc.
Life Changing Books

Library of Congress Catalog Card Number: Registration Filed
ISBN: 0-9764232-1-9

Photography: Rick Busch Photographics, Minneapolis, MN
Cover Design: Bill Sheeler Design, Minneapolis, MN
Graphic Design and Illustration:
Sara Jo Johnson, Roseville, MN and Elizabeth Johnson, Minneapolis, MN
Edited by: Charlene Meadows, Minneapolis, MN

Published by:
River City Press, Inc.
Life Changing Books & Study Guides
4301 Emerson Avenue North
Minneapolis, Minnesota 55412
1-888-234-3559
http://www.rivercitypress.net

Dedication

To every woman who desires to be simply beautiful inside and out;
may you find the real joy that comes from having a relationship with God
and complete acceptance of how He created you.

In loving memory of my mother-in-law, Gini Swanson,
who was a woman of grace and beauty with a faith that blessed many.

Acknowledgements

To my dear husband, Craig, my daughter Kelsey and my son Kyle for their love, tolerance and sense of humor that carried me through.

To Mom who gave me my sense of style and proved that "an ounce of mother is worth a pound of clergy" and to Dad who told me and *showed* me I could do anything if I worked hard enough.

To my extended family for their encouragement and immense support: physically, mentally and spiritually.

To my publisher Bob Wolf, who believed in this project and went above and beyond the call of duty to make it happen (and to Charlene Meadows, my editor, who told him it was worth it).

To the dynamic duo who spent countless hours on the design work and illustrating of this book, Elizabeth Johnson and Sara Jo Johnson. And to Bill Sheeler whose artistic ability and talent turned out a beautiful cover.

To Rick Busch who did an outstanding job on the photography and all the wonderful models who patiently posed: Linda Rehder, Terri Haut, Faye Wendland, Marla Helseth, Crystal Wolf, Sinath Ly, Lisa Kieger, Sue Swanson, Kori Gowan, Tiffany Siems, Alice Wagner, Carol Lundberg, Rosella Cotrone, and Nicole Tombers.

To Susan Titus Osborn for her meticulous job pre-editing.

To my friends Kathy, Debbie, Lesley, Joy, Jeneria, Rita, Cherie and the gals in Coffee and Friends Bible study for giving me emotional and prayer support.

And a special thanks to my dear friend Terri Gardner, who sifted through every page of this book – numerous times, and generously gave of herself to get me through the last few years.

This book was not done alone by my hands, but by the hands and ideas of many people. While I wish I could name everyone, it would be impossible. But you know who you are, and this project could not have come together without your advice, time and prayers. My heartfelt thank you goes out to you all and I pray that God will bless each one of you in a special way for your contribution here.

CONTENTS

INTRODUCTION

What should I wear? This question epitomized the story of my life—*literally.* As a teenager, dressing for school began with a rigorous morning of fashion show calisthenics. The warm-up involved great uncertainty as I pulled countless articles of clothing out of my closet, creating and changing outfits at least three times before dashing out the door. But it didn't end there; many times I'd race back to the bedroom to make a wardrobe adjustment before it was show time, and I would end up missing the bus. This set the stage for my life's career.

Today, twenty-five years later, as a professional image consultant, I stand before my hanging textile collection and contemplate the day's clothing strategy. Only now am I tactically more confident and efficient. After years of sifting through clothes that included, "the good, the bad, and the ugly," the outfits that have survived help me make peace with my ever-changing body. As we all learn, I have become sorely aware that gravity is not my friend and oft a powerful contender in the enemy ranks.

Over the last two decades I have advised thousands of women ages 18-89 on fashion and color ideas from hairstyles to heels. They come in with questions like: "Can I wear black?" "How can I hide my thunder thighs?" or, "What lipstick should I use?" After the consultation they leave with a clearer understanding of how to flatter their figure, enhance their features, and have a better appreciation for the body they've been blessed with.

God is the artistic Creator who has designed each of us as His own unique masterpiece. My job is to instruct how to best frame that picture within the context of clothing, color, and cosmetics. The real reward in my work comes from the positive self-image that begins to emerge in the client who has made a choice to change what she can and gracefully accept what she cannot. There is a glow of self-confidence that becomes apparent as she starts to make new choices with her clothing and makeup with greater ease than ever before.

Robert Browning once said, "If you get simple beauty and nought else, you get about the best thing God invents." My purpose in writing this book is to teach women the art of "simple beauty."

May you find yourself on a journey of renewal and contentment as you discover the beauty God has created in you and recognize the importance of nurturing the "unfading beauty" referred to in the Bible—that which will last far beyond what this life has to offer.

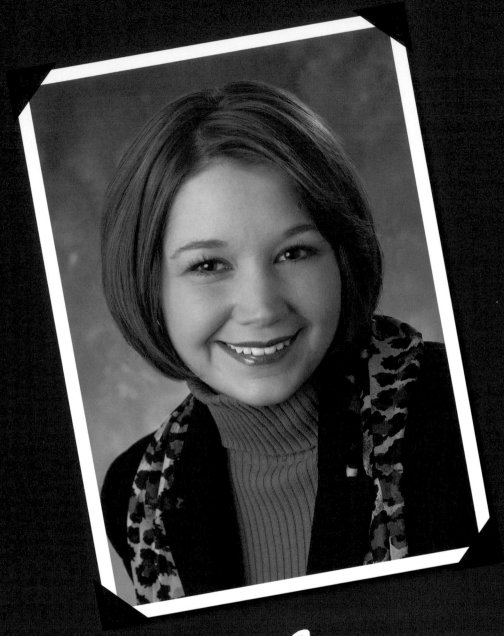

Simply Beautiful

BEAUTY WITHOUT **1** VANITY

Balancing beauty with humility is an on-going struggle for today's woman. None of us want to appear vogue on the outside and vague on the inside. If we were to be honest with ourselves, we would all like to look the best we can. Clothing and appearance affect how we feel and think about ourselves. They can lift our spirits and help give us confidence to face the real world.

The body is God's handiwork. We have a responsibility to take care of it and to present ourselves in a way that will compliment the Kingdom of God. How we appear on the outside reflects our integrity and competence. In our initial contact with people, fifty-five percent of our perceived credibility is based on appearance alone! First impressions lay the groundwork for establishing trust and believability.

■ Dressed to Express

If we are to be salt and light in a world where man judges by outward appearances, then we need to move forward and make some changes. Though clothes do not make the person, we often become what we wear. When we embrace an outer image that dates us, people think our ideas and opinions are dated as well.

If a woman came to your door offering expertise on interior decorating dressed in a frumpy polyester suit, bouffant hairdo, and oversized glasses, would you be willing to hire her to redesign your domain? Probably not. What if she wanted to share her spiritual beliefs? Most of us would make up an excuse for why we couldn't listen at that time or politely say no. Now imagine that same woman with an updated hairstyle and glasses, dressed in a structured black suit with a crisp white blouse. Suddenly, she has our attention and respect! This ensemble communicates power and professionalism. What we look like can instill confidence and influence how we are perceived by others.

Often people lock themselves into a comfortable time and space capsule as if change represents a loss of "mastery" over conquered elements and a mournful departure of youth and happiness. These individuals clingingly hold to what they perceive as security and close the door to opportunity and all the good things that time brings. Change can be painful, even if it is good, and especially if it is happening to us.

I had a client who came into my office for a complete "before and after" makeover. Janet had been wearing the same hairstyle for quite some time. It was reminiscent of the Farrah Fawcett look made popular in the late 70's. Her makeup consisted of a beautiful smile and some occasional mascara, while her "comfortable" wardrobe camouflaged her shapely figure.

When I called to confirm her appointment, she was on the verge of backing out. "I don't think I can go through with this. My stomach is in knots, and I tossed and turned all night." I assured her it would be worthwhile and gently reminded her that now was the time for change. While her style remained dormant, her body, life, and personality had not.

Janet did make it into my office that day, and after a new haircut, makeup, and wardrobing tips, she went home relieved with a glow on her face that mirrored the sparkle in her personality. I received a letter from her shortly after saying, "I am a new woman!" In the closing of the letter, she thanked me and admitted, "Change is good."

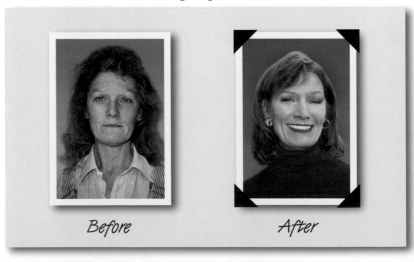

Before   *After*

John Wesley, the 18th Century evangelist, put it best when he said, "As to matters of dress, I would recommend one never to be the first in the fashion nor the last out of it."

Dressed to Excess

Another major fashion problem encountered by women in all walks of life is an over-abundance of clothing, accessories, and beauty products, not to mention lack of time. Many of us have swallowed the idea that the more clothes we amass, the more outfits we'll have and the better we will look. This is deception at its best. On the surface is the appearance of logic (this piece will go with everything), but the reality is somewhere far beneath. Slowly, we women hunt and gather our fabric treasures, storing and saving, bagging and boxing, folding and hanging, until one day we open the doors and drawers to find fragments of disassociated and discombobulated pieces and parts. Truth is, too much of anything complicates life.

Women today want to make the most of what they've got, do it effortlessly every day, and be able to forget about it. The problem stems from our habit of believing "more is better." The solution? *Simplification.* Ultimately, tackling the closet, streamlining the wardrobe, and fast-forwarding the beauty routine allows more time and energy to concentrate on the qualities within ourselves that contribute to God's purpose for our lives.

The secrets for getting dressed at a moment's notice and looking polished and put together with ease lie in the pages ahead. You will discover how to evaluate, eliminate, and accentuate your personal style and wardrobe, making your beauty routine less complicated and your life easier. I will share with you **simple** ways to:

- ☐ Use color and style to refine and define your natural beauty.
- ☐ Apply makeup for a fast, fabulous face.
- ☐ Learn how to organize your closet and alleviate "dressing and stressing."
- ☐ Update, accessorize, and shop wise.
- ☐ Color your attitude with unfading beauty that will last beyond this life.

Join me in an endeavor to enhance our beauty both inside and out, freeing us to go forth, *"Therefore, as God's chosen people, holy and dearly loved, clothe yourselves with compassion, kindness, humility, gentleness and patience." (Colossians 3:12)*

■ The Simplicity of "1"

Dressing would be easier if we could just go back to the "good ol' days" when each woman had one coat, one pair of shoes, one dress for church, and a pair of overalls for everything else. You never had to fret over what to wear or fear that your purchases would make you a fashion misfit by becoming obsolete in a few short months.

We ascribe beauty to that which is simple.
—Ralph Waldo Emerson

The agony of making decisions about the major purchases within our closets can be emotionally and financially draining. About the time we think we've got it all together in our closet, one glance at the latest fashion magazine screams that the trend has already changed. Colors that were "the rage" are now passé. Hem-lengths have moved down the leg three inches, and all those low-rise slacks that replaced the old basics last year are nowhere to be seen. How defeating! While fashion today offers an abundance of choices, the rules and changes it dictates lure us into buying more than is really necessary to suit our varied lifestyles.

This chapter holds the keys to enabling us to make wise choices on the core clothing pieces and accessories needed to build a wardrobe. "Simplicity of 1" is the secret formula to making our apparel needs more manageable. These techniques will save time and money while shopping and help us make everyday color decisions easily. As we learn to use these concepts, we will be free to focus more on the things we like to shop for—the unique pieces that characterize our personal style.

Some have a signature style that is defined by accessories such as flamboyant scarves, multiple bracelets, or a slew of shoes. One client of mine has a passion for hats. Lisa has one in almost every color, shape and texture. She enjoys not only wearing and shopping for them, but displaying them as well. It's who she is, the "hat lady," and Lisa's unique fedoras add intriguing insight to her character during first impressions.

There are women who collect specific designer clothes, and others with single-color compulsions where 90 percent of what's in the closet is primarily one color (usually black). There are even those who accumulate coats—like me. My rationale is that living in a cold climate, a coat is the article of clothing most people see nine months out of the year anyway. I have a variety of colors, shapes, and designs, and delight in wearing each one.

Whether you choose to justify your guilty pleasure or revel in it, there are other areas you can scale down to make more room for your signature style pieces. As we learn to work with our God-given coloring, we discover shortcuts we can take to streamline our everyday wardrobe needs, thereby giving us a basic core to our closets. We start with the "bare essentials"—simple basic pieces to anchor our look with ease.

Choose rather to want less than to have more.
—Thomas A. Kempis

The Essential Shoes

Have you ever passed up wearing a flattering outfit from your closet simply because you didn't have the right shoes to go with it? Wouldn't it be nice to discover a way to eliminate some of those extra pairs of shoes that are collecting dust? Well, consider this:

One to two pairs of shoes can coordinate with 80 percent of the clothes you own

If you have a "fetish for footwear" or are a "colossal collector of shoes," you may want to skip this section. Then again, it may inspire you to buy one more pair….

Pairing Down

Start by choosing a hosiery color that looks natural with your skin tone or one shade darker (taupe, cocoa, beige, suntan, or nude). Wear these hose the next time you are shoe shopping. The goal is to find a simple, classic shoe that blends in with the color of your nylon-clad legs (pumps with a two to three inch heel are recommended). The closer the color match, the better. Don't skimp on comfort – these are shoes you will wear out. Invest wisely.

Next, try these shoes with the existing clothes in your wardrobe and see how many outfits they actually complement. The neutral shoes, provided they are comfortable and look good on your feet, will get worn far more often than any other pair you own.

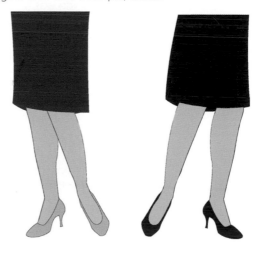

Matching your shoe and leg color will make your legs appear visibly longer, and the longer they look, the slimmer they look.

This tip works particularly well with skirts and dresses.

When you wear your red shoes with your red dress (as fashion dictates you should), people will notice your shoes. While that may be appropriate for bridesmaids, it's costly when you are dealing with the contents of your closet (to say nothing of the fact that if you have large feet, it makes them the show piece). When the shoe matches the leg, the shoe color goes unnoticed because the eye stops at the hemline, and nothing calls attention to the feet.

Carry this idea through the warmer months by getting a pair of sandals that match your bare feet. Shorts, skirts, dresses, and even slacks will coordinate easily with footwear that blends. Keep this in mind when traveling. There is a lot less bulk when you have only one or two pair of shoes in the suitcase.

Your second pair of shoes should be very dark brown or black, whichever you wear more of in your wardrobe. Get a pair made from quality materials and stick with a simple style.

The Essential Purse

It has been said that a woman's purse is her "flash of success." When we throw our bag over our shoulder, it's there for everyone to see. It tells a tale of the lifestyle we lead and can either make or break our look.

Martha was the quintessential "bag" lady. When I first saw this petite woman in her early fifties, I thought she was a professional weight lifter. Because the size of her purse was one-third the size of her body, I concluded that the muscle required to carry such a suitcase must involve some serious strength training. It overwhelmed her small frame and made her look like a door-to-door salesperson on call 24/7. We assessed the contents of the bag and discovered that most of the items could be eliminated or stored in her car's glove compartment. Finding a smaller purse that was functional and fashionable put a new spring into Martha's step.

While some enjoy the sport of switching purses to coordinate with each ensemble, many of us stay with the old tried-and-true to conserve time and energy. To simplify one's life, let us consider the "essential purse."

There are three key elements in choosing a good purse:

- ■ Appearance ■ Function ■ Quality

■ Appearance

A purse color is most stylish when it matches the shoe color. When the handbag sits on the floor it will *blend* with what's on the feet. For your everyday purse, follow the lead of the "essential shoe" matching your leg color. When it is hanging on the shoulder, it will meld into the rest of the outfit.

A second color choice for a purse would be a shade that blends with your hair color. This will lead the eye up to your face and look natural with the rest of your coloring. Another option is to select a dark neutral, black or brown.

Try the purse on. Is it the right size? If you have a larger frame and carry a purse that is too small, it will make you look proportionally larger. If you are petite and carry a large bag, it can overpower your look. Scale the bag to your size and height.

Observe where the purse hangs on your body: Is it in a "positive or negative" area?

If you have heavy hips or thighs, a bag resting at the same level will add extra weight there. The same results apply if you have extra inches around your waist and the purse hangs near the midriff. Put the purse on your shoulder and lift the top of the strap to position it at different heights. If the strap is too long, have it shortened; adjustments can be made by a shoe repair shop.

■ Function

Function means having a purse that suits your lifestyle. Does it allow you to find things easily? Keep the compartments to a minimum. The more zippers and pockets, the more time wasted looking for things. One or two zippers are plenty.

How many steps does it take to retrieve money from your purse? 1) Lift flap. 2) Unzip zipper. 3) Take out wallet. 4) Unsnap wallet. 5) Open wallet…. Why not select a one-step flap purse with a place for all your credit cards and money under it?

An outside pocket on the purse allows for easy accessibility to sunglasses, keys, or lists. Reserve a spot in that pocket for a pen. A leather repair shop can stitch a seam down one end of the pocket an inch from the edge to accommodate a pen in an upright position.

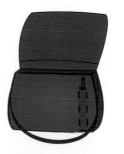

Another option is to have a loop sewn inside to slide a pen into a convenient spot.

Are you a mother who carries a diaper bag *and* a purse? Scale down when possible to either a large classy purse, roomy enough for a diaper and disposable wipes, or a small wallet-style purse with a strap to tuck into the diaper bag.

◼ Quality

Consider your everyday purse as a "personal tool bag." It is used 365 days a year, and your organized life centers around its contents. I recommend buying the best purse you can afford. It will upgrade an outfit and improve your image. Quality leather and workmanship are a must. Are the seams stitched evenly and tightly? Is the hardware brass or plastic? Do the zippers and closures work with ease?

How much is it worth to you to have a hassle-free handbag? At ten cents a day, for two years, a $73 investment can prove to be a wise choice. If you are considering a higher-end option, a classic Coach (Coach, Inc. Manhattan, NY) bag will cost considerably more, but will last five years with good care. This company also has a warranty on the stitching, binding, and hardware in its products.

Regardless of the choice you make, keep the style simple. The less detail, the classier it will appear, and the better it will retain that look. And finally, keep your purse clean. A dirty purse makes your entire appearance dowdy.

◼ The Essential Coat

Having one coat that will coordinate with whatever is worn beneath it is as easy as looking in the mirror. Take a good look at the colors in your hair and select a coat that matches one of the dominant shades. This technique has been used for years in fur sales when helping people choose a pelt that will look fabulous with anything. The coat will blend and look like it belongs on the wearer. With this in mind, I also strongly recommend that a bright-colored scarf and/or hat be added to enhance the face. Your best accent color would be your lip color or your eye color (if it is something other than your hair color).

Quality is important. Your everyday coat is the one piece of clothing that more people see on you in public than anything else you own. Figure in your "cost per wearing" when deciding if you are spending too much for this article. Choose high-quality fabric and construction.

Make comfort and efficiency a priority. How easy does it slide over your clothes? Do you have a free range of movement? Does it bind? Is it too heavy? You want something that is comfortable and wearable on a daily basis.

Keep the style simple and details to a minimum. The essential coat will serve you well in the years to come.

Let's face it, the "good ol' days" were practical but also dull and uninspiring. Variety is fun, and the "Simplicity of 1" is not meant to limit your personal style. If you are a "shoe horse," saddle up, have a ball, and buy them all! You can always save money and closet space in the purse or coat category with this theory. The goal is to have peace of mind in knowing that you have something that works with whatever you choose to wear and to free you from being a slave to fashion.

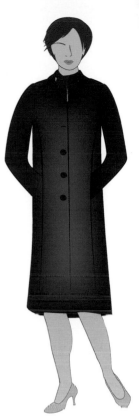

■ Making Wise the Simple

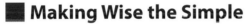

The key to keeping life simple is recognizing what is essential to our lives and what is not. Learning to establish our priorities based on God's purpose for us will give direction when planning our days, spending our money, or setting our goals. What is to be our top priority? *To "seek first His kingdom and His righteousness." (Matthew 6:33a)* It begins with a simple faith: believing and behaving.

A mountain climber fell off a cliff while out hiking. Fortunately, he was able to grab a branch on the way down. Hanging on for dear life, he began yelling, "Help! Help! Is anyone there?" A voice responded, "I am here and I will save you if you believe in me." The man yelled back, "I believe! I believe!" The voice replied, "If you believe in me, let go of the branch, and I will save you." The man looked down at the rocks below and looked back up and said, "Is there anyone else up there?" Faith means we must trust and obey.

How do we get faith? Romans 10:17 says:

"Consequently, faith comes from hearing the message, and the message is heard through the Word of Christ."

We need to consistently read our Bibles. Spending time with and listening to another person is the best way to get to know someone. Having a relationship builds trust that results in faith. Sometimes we fall into the habit of carrying on a one-sided conversation with God by praying and neglecting to open our Bibles and listening to His ideas.

Reading God's Word and understanding it can be a spiritual challenge. Start with a prayer asking for the Holy Spirit's guidance as you read. The Bible is the only book you can read every time with the author looking over your shoulder. It becomes an interactive tool as God directs our attention and enlightens us in our specific areas of need.

A simple way to get the most out of each passage is to use the S.T.O.P. technique. Read a short segment, stop, and ask yourself:

STOP

Is there something here I need to:

be SORRY for?

be THANKFUL for?

be OBEDIENT for?

or PRAY for?

Meditating on God's Word keeps our perspective in check and helps us deal with daily struggles and stress. Our faith and relationship with Jesus will grow stronger as we study this manual for life, the B.I.B.L.E. – Basic Instructions Before Leaving Earth.

7 SIMPLE STEPS

1. List two things you would like to change about yourself physically:

   _____

   _____

2. Set two goals for yourself for spiritual growth:

   _____

   _____

3. Begin looking for the essential coat.

4. Choose a neutral color of hose and a pair of shoes to match.

5. Sort out the contents of your purse, evaluate and eliminate.

6. List the top three priorities in your life:

   _____

   _____

   _____

7. Write: S.T.O.P. on a slip of paper and place it in your Bible as a bookmarker.

   STOP

   Is there something here I need to:

   be SORRY for?

   be THANKFUL for?

   be OBEDIENT for?

   or PRAY for?

Simply Beautiful

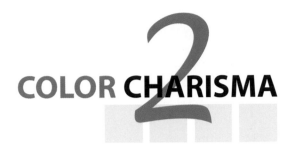

COLOR CHARISMA

First impressions are lasting impressions—it's a well-publicized fact. However, did you know that when someone first meets you, they remember approximately ninety percent of what you look like and only ten percent of what you say? Of that ninety percent, the key thing a person will recall is color-related: The color of our clothing, skin, and hair.

Over the years, I have become acutely aware of this. After pouring my heart and soul into a speech, three months later, I encountered an audience member who said, "Oh, I heard you speak last spring at the auxiliary luncheon. I remember because you had on such a beautiful coral suit that day." So much for my articulate words and enlightening presentation. The truth is, little is ever remembered about the content. It's the visual aspect that leaves the most lasting impression.

▉ Signature Colors

The foundation to building your own best look originates in one's personal "signature colors." They are the cornerstones that create a harmonious relationship within your closet to combine colors and develop a wardrobe that enhances your features. These flattering colors will also give you the freedom and ease to wear *any* color successfully.

Signature colors are the shades that reflect and advance our own natural coloring. They are what we see when we look into a mirror; the key is to copy what you see. A royal blue blouse worn by a woman with bright blue eyes will spark countless comments on how the color flatters her eyes. A child with dark hair and rosy lips dressed in red will gain attention and compliments throughout the day. The power of signature colors is in their ability to captivate an individual's unique attributes and implant that impression in another person's mind by making a visual connection between two matching colors.

The three prominent signature colors are:

1. **Eye Color** — Your eye color is the most convincing color you have when communicating one-on-one. If you want a person to listen to you and believe what you have to say, wear the color of your eyes in a shirt or accessory near your face. You will have them looking directly into your eyes, and when you maintain eye contact, you achieve better communication skills.

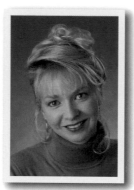

This periwinkle sweater brings out Sue's beautiful eyes and complements the cool tones in her skin color.

2. **Lip Color** — Wearing a blouse that matches your lip color will bring a beautiful healthy glow to your face and a day filled with compliments. It is one of the most attractive colors you can choose for a blouse or sweater. When you are feeling under the weather, it will perk up your look and restore color to your cheeks. A shirt or sweater in your lipstick color is also an excellent option if you plan to get your picture taken.

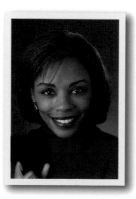

Marla's elegant and understated beauty is dazzling particularly when accented with red in her lip color and turtleneck sweater.

3. **Hair Color** — The perfect neutral shade for a suit or coat is your hair color. When choosing this color, be certain to get it in an interesting fabric. As a general rule, the duller the color, the more luxurious the fabric should be. Therefore, tones of grays, browns, and beiges need extra help. Note: When possible, use an accent color near your face such as a bright scarf or shirt color.

Belts, purses, and shoes in shades of your hair color will work well for most of your casual outfits.

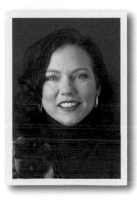

The warm tones in Crystal's rich brown hair are further enhanced with the chocolate shade of her sweater.

Keep in mind that any time you wear a color similar to one of your features, it will draw attention to that area. If you wear your hair color when having a bad hair day, be cautious because people *will* notice your hair!

Some of us have hair and eye colors that are almost identical (brown for example), adding more impact to that color when you wear it. People with a combination of colors in their hair or eyes have a broader spectrum of signature colors to choose from. A brunette with auburn highlights can look wonderful in a russet or brown tweed jacket. Flecks of yellow in blue eyes will add interesting tones of aqua and turquoise to their palate. People with green-brown eyes may find a deep olive sweater very complementary to their coloring.

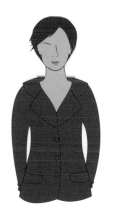

Giving New Life to Your Wardrobe

Combining signature colors with the unflattering shades in one's closet will resuscitate a wardrobe, making tired pieces wearable. For example: A charcoal gray suit produces a pale, washed-out cast to my own skin tone. When paired with a coral blouse that complements my lip color, it makes me look alive! Add to that blouse gray pearl buttons and it bridges the gap— creating an attractive color combination.

Other unique blends include red and brown, rose and olive, aqua and purple, or black and caramel pictured here on Tiffany. She knows that black isn't her best color, however the warm tone in the turtleneck matches her eyes and hair. Using an animal print scarf to accessorize the ensemble pulls the outfit together and makes her look radiant in an otherwise mediocre color. (The following sections will provide more ideas in this area.)

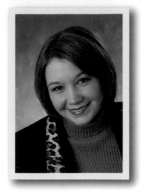

Image Impact

The dress code for leaving a lasting impression is to wear signature colors. For job interviews they will mix effectively with neutrals like black, navy, tan, and gray. If it's an audition you're up for, try a single-color outfit in a raspberry or russet shade that complements your lips. Then, use unique fabrics and textures that vary to add interest (i.e. wool with satin or a sand-washed silk with suede). The person you are trying to impress will notice your features and recall what you looked like long after you walk out of the room.

The stronger the contrast you wear, the more authoritative you appear.

Build a wardrobe around three core colors:

1. **Your Power Color** — This is the color that gives <u>you</u> a strong sense of confidence and boldness when you wear it. For some, a power color is black or navy, others may choose brown or gray—whatever works for you.

2. **Your Favorite Color** — What color do you just love and can't seem to get enough of in your closet? When you wear this color, it will lift your spirits and set your mood for the day.

3. **Your Compliment Color** — Which color do you receive the most compliments on when you wear it? Buy it in a shirt, sweater, *and* jacket and you will get a good return on your investment.

Using your signature colors effectively will give you complete confidence in knowing that your first impression is the lasting impression you desire!

◼ Color Connections

Colors infuse your wardrobe with *life*. While it's one thing to know what shades to wear, combining them in outfits can pose an entirely new challenge. Using colors in unconventional ways will stimulate visual appeal and revive mundane garments. By following a few simple rules, blending shades can add creativity and class to any closet.

1. Combine Unevenly

When a decorator designs a room, there is one dominant color and less of a secondary shade. A third color may be used in a small amount as an "accent." This technique can also be applied in putting an outfit together. A navy blue suit, white shirt, and a fuchsia scarf provide an attractive balance of color. However, a navy jacket, white shirt, and red slacks each compete for attention.

The uneven rule also applies when using two colors: one should be visibly dominant. An ivory skirt and a pink blouse with pearl earrings and necklace create an engaging combination. The pearl accessories pull the lower color up to the face, causing the ivory to prevail.

When using a third color to accentuate an outfit, reinforce it by placing it in two areas. This makes the accent look intentional and not like an after-thought. Position them in close proximity of each other on either the upper or lower half of the body. For example, a royal blue scarf with coordinating earrings, a leopard print purse with matching shoes, or a silver choker with a silver chain belt. Do **not** scatter the accent color throughout your ensemble, or you will look like an argument between competing colors, such as: A blue dress with red shoes, red belt, and red necklace and earrings.

2. Use Elements that Unify

Wearing two unlikely colors together can be harmonious if you know the ties that bind. A coral red suit with a butter-yellow blouse will gain instant approval by replacing the plain matching buttons on the jacket with brushed gold buttons that mimic the yellow shade.

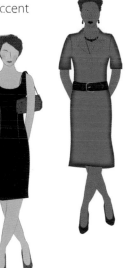

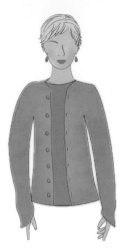

Another way to combine existing wardrobe pieces is to modify accessories. Use nail enamel to change the color and character of jewelry. Pewter coin-shaped earrings, painted with a dash of bright pink polish, will pull together a charcoal sweater and rose T-shirt with finesse.

Patterned scarves provide inspiration for combining unique colors, adding variety and unity to any closet. Try holding a printed scarf at eye-level and slowly walking through your closet, moving it across the clothing. Notice how the garments draw out different colors in the scarf. This expands the possibilities of color combinations not considered before and creates new options for old and rarely worn pieces.

3. Find New Inspirations

Many times we fall back into letting "fashion" dictate our color combinations. Whatever is in style for the season tends to be the trend for blending—whether it is combining the conservative black and white, or a bizarre mix of orange and pink. Start seeking new avenues for inspiring ideas. Look at what is being mixed and matched in the home décor world.

Cool colors like blue and purple make us appear smaller.

That crimson and cream plaid couch accented with spring green pillows may serve to motivate you to put a green vest with your red gingham shirt.

Go to an art gallery and observe the shades and intensities combined in beautiful paintings. Or, simply take a walk outside and see how God does it: green and pink in the flowers, a sunset with oranges and violets, or the vast array of greens in the landscape. This should not only renew your appreciation for nature but also give new insight for fresh combinations of colors.

4. Discover the Magic of Monochromatics

Color can be your closet's best friend or worst enemy. There are times when an elegant statement can only be made with a single color costume. Professionally speaking, the fewer colors you wear the more credible you will appear. Not only does this look sharp, it also gives a lean line to any figure. Using different shades of the same color can also have a strong impact. The key is to use a variety of textures when working with the same or similar hues in an outfit. For instance, a cream sweater, tan suede vest, and camelhair slacks will produce a pleasing combination. Try to keep the lighter shade on the top or at the neckline to highlight the face.

The softer the contrast you have on, the more approachable you appear.

5. Complement Your Contrast

The natural contrast between your hair color and skin tone sets the stage for the intensity of colors that can be worn together most successfully. A woman with dark brown hair and fair skin will benefit by combining light colors with dark ones near her face, such as black and light pink. Two light colors worn together on a brunette will look faded out. The blonde with an ivory complexion will do better with light to medium color combinations, such as a soft yellow and periwinkle blue. Those with dark hair and skin will find that very light or dark colors worn with bright, clear colors are most complementary, such as charcoal gray and bright red. The person with medium hair and skin tone will benefit most by blending medium and dark or medium and light colors accented by a vibrant shade near the face.

The idea is to achieve harmony with your personal coloring, so that *you* are the focus and not the outfit. If a color combination works, it enhances your features and does not call attention to itself. The compliments you hear shouldn't be, "I love that dress," but rather, "You look terrific!"

Understanding how to mix colors is the basis for building a useful wardrobe that is both interesting and flattering. The methods introduced here will not only give you more ideas to work with, but also put to use some of the single and rarely-worn items you've not been able to wear.

■ Color's Silent Language

Color talks and color communicates! Before we even open our mouths the colors we wear can speak volumes about us. The color you are wearing right now can be influencing your mood, how you feel about yourself and how you interact with others. Yet more importantly, not only is it having an effect on you, but also each person you encounter.

Using color correctly can add credibility and confidence. For instance, an outfit with red in it, worn to a job interview, will not only build self-assurance, but research has found it gives a competitive edge in landing the job. You appear more energetic and capable of handling whatever comes your way.

Incorrect use of color can cause miscommunications or in some cases actually undermine our mission. For example, if a substitute teacher walks into a junior high classroom wearing a pink shirt and a lavender suit, she will establish a mood for the room before uttering a word. While a few of the gentler students may view her as kind and approachable, the vast majority of the class will see her as a pushover. Unless she is six-foot-four and built like a pro wrestler, this lady is going to have one long and difficult day. By contrast, if she arrives in a black suit and white shirt, the kids will not be able to detect her disposition because black conceals the personality of the individual wearing it, and the look will command respect before using any verbal communication.

Try the color cream instead of black for a dressy and classy evening look.

Color can be used to express oneself, conveying a message more effectively. It has been said that in order to establish trust and credibility, seven percent is what you say, thirty-eight percent is how you say it, and fifty-five percent is what you looked like when you said it. Color is the first thing a person notices about you and the last thing they remember.

Defining the Hues

Generally speaking, color can be quickly defined by looking at two factors: intensity and depth.

Intensity

Brighter colors advance. People tend to believe the brighter the color (red, orange, yellow), the more outgoing the personality is. A muted color, such as gray, brown, and beige, tends to represent a more reserved nature.

Bright

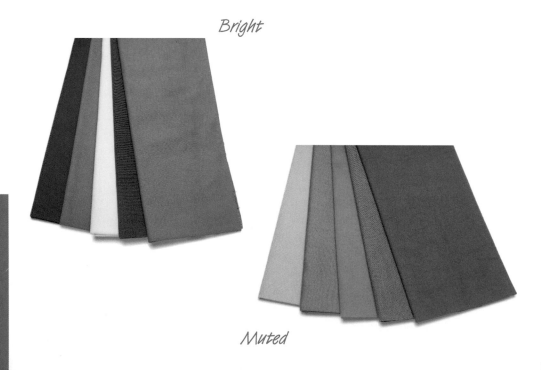

Muted

▨ Depth

Dark colors like black, charcoal, and navy, project strength, authority, and drama. Light colors come across as approachable, friendly, and gentle, for example: light pink, baby blue, and peach.

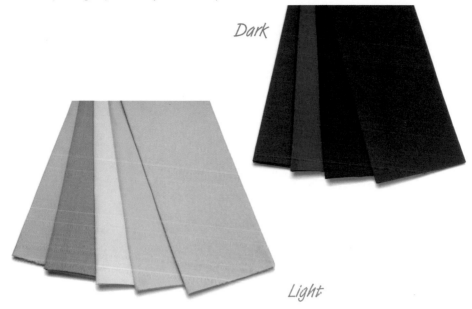

Dark

Light

If you want to be left alone for the day, wear yellow and black. They represent "warning colors" in nature such as the bumble bee and in society as seen in caution signs.

The following is a simple guideline to aid you in understanding the meanings behind some of the basic colors we use in our wardrobes. This information has been derived from years of research including the insights of authors Leatrice Eiseman, *Alive with Color*, and Carlton Wagner who wrote *Color Power*.

Color Dictionary

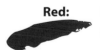

Red: Demands attention; shows power, confidence, energy, and courage; attracts and excites.

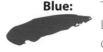

Blue: Trustworthy and dependable; calming and approachable. Light blue: kind and serene. Dark blue: respectable, conservative, and intelligent.

Yellow: Radiates joy and attracts attention; people oriented, and optimistic; gives you, as well as others, an emotional lift.

Green: Emotionally calming; stable, down-to-earth, loyal and hard-working; nurturing and helpful.

Orange: Attracts people, fun and energetic, extrovert; adventurer.

Violet: Creative and sensitive. Dark purple: individualist, mysterious, self-confident. Lavender: romantic.

Pink: Approachable, gentle, kind and compassionate, charitable and loving.

Brown: A good listener who puts others at ease, stimulates conversation; secure but not haughty, humble, supportive.

Gray: Denotes a strong work ethic: passive, mature, efficient, wise, refined.

Black: Authoritative, sophisticated and respectable; independent, intimidating, intriguing.

White: Clean, refined and open to change; purity, innocence, and morality; inspires trust.

The key is to learn to choose color not only in terms of what looks good on you, but also consider the response it will generate. Learn to use color to your advantage, both physically and emotionally. How a color feels can be more important than how a color looks.

■ Color Me True

When I first began my business, twenty-three years ago, having one's colors done was "the rage." Being an image consultant was a highly competitive field, and I worked hard to stay on top of things. The popular book "*Color Me Beautiful*" had just been released, and one of their analysts booked a presentation at a local church in our city. I wanted to hear her speech but was concerned that someone would recognize me and question my presence. So I devised a plan to go incognito.

Slicking my hair back into a tight bun, I put on some large glasses, and wore a lavender maternity smock. To complete the costume I strapped a large pillow around my waist and positioned it front and center so I looked like I was well into my ninth month of pregnancy. Since I'd never been pregnant, I spent the afternoon practicing the waddle walk and slowly sitting down in chairs as I had observed my expectant friends do.

By evening I was ready. I arrived early at the church and found an empty table in the back. I sat there with a sense of devious confidence until three women came and joined me—three *pregnant* women. I knew I was in trouble when they gleefully tried to engage me in conversation. "Is this your first?" I swallowed hard, "Uh, yes." "Who is your OBGYN?" "My who?" "What trimester are you in?" "Trimester?" My heart raced as I tried to talk the talk after I had "walked the walk." It reminded me of the Proverb: "*Even a fool is thought wise if he keeps silent*" (17:28a). It proved to be a very long evening.

Since man looks at the outward appearance, it's easy to fool people into believing we are something we may not be, that is until we open our mouths. Can someone judge that you are a Christian by the way you talk? What do you color your words with? Is it consistent with who you are at home? Or are you like me on a stressful day, screaming at the kids one minute and answering the phone the next with a sweet and perky, "Hello!" masquerading as a cheerful, Spirit-filled woman of God?

According to the Bible, *kindness* makes a man attractive. (Proverbs 19:22a TLB) Before you open your mouth, test what you are about to say. Ask: Is it kind? Is it true? And, is it necessary? When you feel the nudging to keep quiet, obey. The Holy Spirit is helping you, do not quench Him, instead, quench your words.

Do not let any unwholesome talk come out of your mouths, but only what is helpful for building others up according to their needs, that it may benefit those who listen. (Ephesians 4:29)

7 SIMPLE STEPS

1. Choose a suit or blazer in your "power color."

2. Find a blouse or shirt that is your "compliment color."

3. Buy a comfortable sweatshirt in your "favorite color."

4. Combine two new colors in your wardrobe and use an accessory or detail to finish off the look.

5. Wear a color that speaks for you to help generate a positive response in relating to others.

6. Have your colors analyzed by a professional Image consultant. It will be the best money you ever spent on yourself.

7. Think before you speak and ask: Is it true? Is it kind? And, is it necessary? Pray that God will use your mouth to encourage and bless others each day.

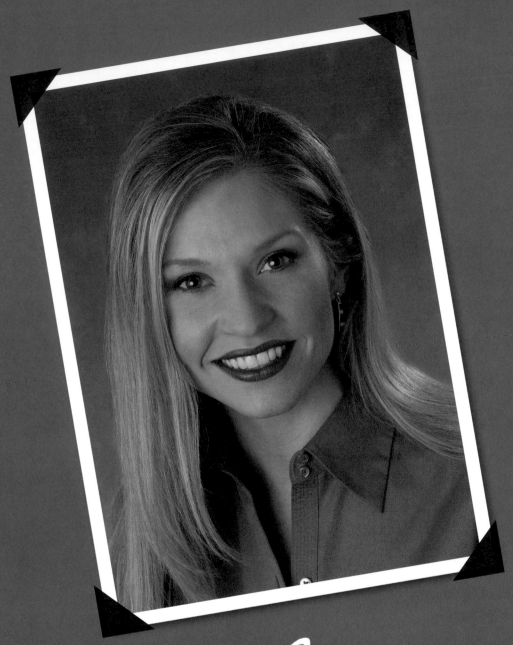

Simply Beautiful

MAKEUP MADE SIMPLE
3

"A little bit of paint on the side of the barn never hurt anything."

I first heard this phrase sitting on a church pew in a small Midwest town, as the German minister leaned over his pulpit and began his sermon. I don't recall exactly what the message was about, but I never forgot the impact that one little sentence had on me.

Too often women are quick to criticize each other's attempts to apply a little paint. For some, wearing cosmetics is not an option as they fear appearing too overdone or being ridiculed. For others, it's simply a lack of time and general know-how.

The point I believe the pastor was trying to communicate was two-fold. First, that we should not judge another because they wear makeup and second, that *a little bit of paint* won't hurt any of us. In other words, make the most of what you've got and keep quiet about other's decisions to do so!

The intent of this chapter is to help you simplify your make-up routine and give guidelines and information about products and techniques to enhance your *natural* beauty.

Basic Cosmetics 101

Wouldn't it be nice to get down to having only one lipstick, one blush, and one shade of nail enamel? While I admit that adjusting lip color to accommodate the shade of an outfit is an attractive plus, most of us don't care to haul around six tubes of lipstick and three blushes to achieve this look. So, find your best and lose the rest.

Beautifying your face can easily be accomplished in as little as five to fifteen minutes. The goal is to present a polished and fresh look. Let's start out with the basics:

Foundation

Purpose: To even out the overall color and smooth the texture of the skin. Some women look fantastic without it, others can look ten years younger by giving it a try.

Product: Foundations come in a variety of formulas including: liquids, creams and solid forms. For a light coverage try a water-based liquid (this can be thinned further by mixing a dab of foundation on your fingertip with a drop of water on another finger and then applying it to the face). Choosing a cream foundation with a "whipped" or "mousse" consistency will also give a lighter feel on the skin. For long lasting, full coverage use products that contain silicone, moisture (oil) based liquids or thicker (dense) cream foundations that come in a compact or stick. Powder foundations are great for quick applications but beware: they may tend to cake.

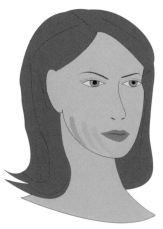

Color: It should match perfectly. The most effective way to achieve this is to try several different colors on your jaw line. Swipe it on, don't blend it in. Allow it to sit for one to two minutes, then look in the mirror. If a color disappears with your skin tone you have it right. If none of them "disappear," proceed to a new set of colors or a different cosmetic line. Remember to buy a deeper shade in summer for slightly tanned skin.

Application: If it's liquid, apply it with fingertips. Dot it on in each quadrant of your face and lightly blend it in evenly. Finish the look by going over your face with a white cosmetic sponge in a downward motion to smooth out the finish. Use the sponge to go on and under the jaw line to prevent "ring around the face." Cream foundations are best applied with a cosmetic sponge in a downward motion.

A face powder can be used to set the makeup that's been applied or also as a base color. If you are inclined to have

Foundation with a moisturizer and SPF built in is a great time saver.

noticeable facial hair, use a minimal amount and avoid the lower cheek and chin area when using a powder product. Powder clings to hair and makes it more pronounced.

Simplify: For a more natural look and easier application, liquid foundations can be thinned down. Water-base: take a small dollop of foundation on the middle finger of one hand and a drop of water on your other middle finger and blending the two together, then apply it to your face. Oil base: thin in the same way using moisturizer instead of water.

Concealer

Purpose: To cover dark shadows around your eye area and other "imperfections."

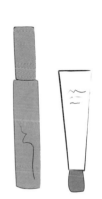

Product: Choose a consistency that works with your skin type. As we age, most of these products will settle into the character lines under our eyes and create a new dilemma. Find a concealer that will cover and not cake.

Color: Match to skin color or go one-half shade lighter. Do not go too light, or you may end up looking like a circus clown.

Application: Apply *sparingly*. In this case, more is not better. Too much will crease and give a wrinkled look around the eye area. Start at the inside corner of the eye next to the nose and put a thin line of color on only the darkest, deepest area. If the concealer does not have an applicator, use a cotton swab. Carefully blend within the dark area using your ring finger (it's weaker and will be easier on the tissue around the eye). Finish it off by smoothing with a cosmetic sponge.

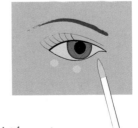

Use a small amount of concealer around the outer eye area, just outside of the "crow's feet." This will give you a youthful glow and brighter eyes.

Simplify: Foundation may also be used in place of concealer if you are looking for a light coverage. A nude color pencil will cover blemishes and can be used in small deep areas you want to lighten up (e.g. around the corner of the nose, or even to soften wrinkles).

After applying makeup study from all angles. The best place is your car's rearview mirror in the natural light.

Eyeliner

Purpose: To define the eye and enhance the lash line, making the eye appear larger.

Product: Liquid liners give a distinct, polished look. Eye pencils will give a softer look.

Color: When working with liquids use neutral shades, such as dark brown, black, or slate. Pencils can be navy, teal, dark green, gray-blue, or dark brown to complement the eye color.

Application: Liquid liner should go on before other eye makeup. Have a damp cotton swab ready to go. Draw the line from the start of the lashes in the inner corner of the eye to the outer end. Immediately use the damp swab to remove the outer thickness of the line. Repeat on bottom lash line.

Pencil: Use a thin pencil and keep it very sharp. Wipe the tip of the pencil with a facial tissue to remove any oil residue. If you have a thick upper lid that is visible with the eye open, line the entire lid. If the eye has an average lid, line from a point in the middle lid to outer edge.

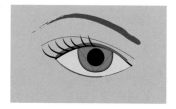

The beginning point of the liner should be very thin. The bottom lid can be lined from the center area out to the edge. Thin pencil liner with a dry swab, taking care not to transfer cotton fibers onto lashes.

Simplify: Try using your powder eyeshadow as a liner by dipping a small thin brush into water then into the shadow color, paint it along the lash line and soften with a cotton swab.

For a quick eye-lift, dab Preparation H gel or cream (not ointment) around eye area, it will minimize lines. A little dab will also shrink pimples!

Mascara

Purpose: To enhance eyelashes, open up the eyes.

Product: It is important that this product is replaced every three months after it's opened (old mascara harbors bacteria that can cause eye infections). The good news is a cheaper brand brings the same results as its expensive counterpart.

Color: Black or dark brown work best. If you want to experiment with a colored mascara, try "mink-tipping." Apply the unique color from base out to the ends of the lashes, then do the tips in brown or black. This will give the illusion of a color liner pencil without the work.

Application: Stroke mascara from base to tip of all lashes. To eliminate clumps, comb through with a metal lash comb (plastic ones do not work well). A second coat can be applied to the outer half of your eyelashes on the top and bottom. This will open up the eye area and make your eyes appear larger. If eyes tear a lot, do not apply mascara to bottom lash line.

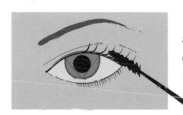

Simplify: If clumping mascara is a chronic problem, use only one coat of color and purchase a new tube of mascara every two months.

Opening your mouth when you apply mascara tightens up the eye area and helps it go on easier.

Eyebrow Color

Purpose: To fill in sparse or thinning eyebrows and complete the "frame" around your eyes.

Product: Available in powder or pencil. Brush-on (powder) brow color looks most natural and is easy to apply. A pencil brow color is quick and convenient.

Color: Choose a shade lighter than your hair color. Brow products tend to go on darker than they appear. Universally, blonde works best for most people. A light brown with a grayish tone also can work well for those with very dark hair. Redheads usually do well with either of these tones and can also experiment with warmer shades.

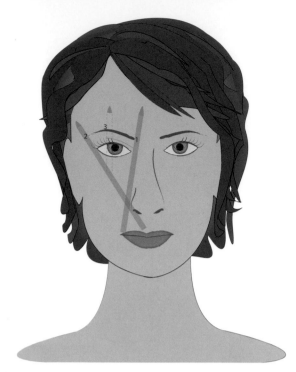

Application: With a pencil use short, wispy strokes to draw in little hairs. Follow the natural line of your brow, or go very slightly higher on the outer ends if they tend to droop down. For boundaries of where to apply the color, use a pencil and follow the guidelines shown here in the illustration. Finish the brows by brushing them backwards with a small brush or toothbrush, then smooth them out with an upward and outward sweep. This will give the illusion of little hairs instead of pencil strokes. Brow color should look natural and not be defined by a solid line.

Simplify: Try a standard sharp #2 pencil for brow color. Many Hollywood makeup artists use this technique.

1) Lay pencil next to nose to find starting point.

2) Lay pencil in corner of nostril and angle up to meet outer corner of eye and brow, this is the ending point.

3) The peak of the brow should line up with the outer edge of the iris.

Eye shadow applied with a stiff brush may also be used as a brow color and is usually easier to match to hair color.

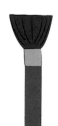

Blush

Purpose: To give a healthy glow and contour to the face.

Product: Cream works well for dry skin types, powder for all skin types, and gel for long-lasting effects.

Color: Gentle shades of pink, rose, peach, and raspberry are all good options *if* they complement your hair and skin tones. If you are unsure, enlist the help of a professional makeup artist or color consultant.

Use a lighter blush for touch-ups to avoid a dark, blotchy look.

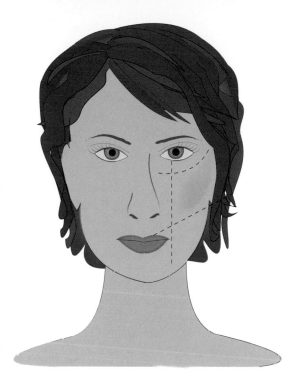

Application: Dab cream blush on with the fingertips just under cheekbone and blend upwards, smoothing out with a sponge. Gels need to be applied quickly and directly to the cheek area where you want the most color (once in place, it won't move). Powders require a good natural-bristle blush brush. Pound bristles of the brush directly down into the blush, then blow the powder into the brush. This will give you a soft color that can be intensified with each stroke.

Simplify: Lipstick may be used as a cream blush. Dot it on the cheek area and blend with fingertips or a sponge.

Lip color

Purpose: To define lips and add color to balance with eyes and hair shades. This will give a finished look to your face, even without other makeup color.

Product:

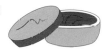

1) Standard matte or creamy consistency in the classic tube works well for everyday.

2) Semi-permanent color is a liquid and dries like nail enamel for longest lasting color.

3) Glosses give temporary shine.

4) Pencils line and color lips.

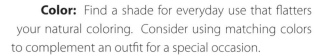

Color: Find a shade for everyday use that flatters your natural coloring. Consider using matching colors to complement an outfit for a special occasion.

Application: Start by lining lips in a pencil shade that matches or is slightly lighter than your lipstick color, following the natural line of your lips. Apply lipstick

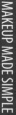

directly from tube (using a lip brush will give a perfected look, but it takes extra time to do).

I suggest steering clear of the neutral brownish shades for lip and cheek color that have gained popularity in recent years. Take a cue from the colors we see in the faces of young children. Rosy lips and natural blush give them their youthful glow. If that were replaced with the beige tones we see in today's lipstick and blush, we would assume the poor child was ill!

For red lipstick without the garish look, apply your everyday lip color and put a dot of the red lipstick in the center of your lips.

Simplify: For long-lasting lip color, use a lip pencil that matches your lipstick not only to line your lips, but to fill in the lip color as well. Then top with lipstick to prevent lips from drying out. Also, powder blush can be used to seal lip color by applying the matching color over lipstick with a cotton swab.

Eye Shadow

Purpose: To complement the eye and its framework, making the eyes the focal point of the face.

Product: Cream for lasting color or powder for ease of application.

Color: Should *complement* the color of your eyes by making eye color stand out, not shadow color. Gone are the days of matching our shadow to our outfit. Choose a neutral highlighter color or base in a light beige or subtle pink. To contour the eye, look for shades that are neutral and nondescript. Gray-brown and gray-purple blend nicely with most eye colors. Brown, green, or hazel eyes can use deep olive.

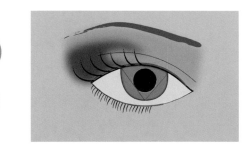

Application: Powder type— Use a sponge tip applicator to apply the highlighter color over the entire lid area. Follow with a layer of darker shadow in a V-shape at the outer corner of eyes to lift. Dust with a soft natural bristle brush blending up and outward.

Cream formulas—use your ring finger to apply light color under brow and on lid. Put dark color just above crease of lid, working from the middle to the outer half of eye.

Simplify: Use pressed powder in place of your eye shadow highlighter color. Apply it to the lid with a sponge applicator. It will match perfectly and be more cost efficient in the long run.

Try mixing eyeshadows together for a more natural, subtle color (ex. brown and green or gray and blue).

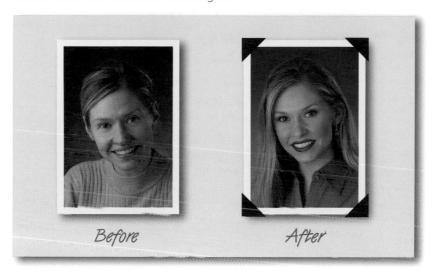

Before   After

Kori is a natural beauty with an artistic talent for applying her own makeup. We chose colors to give her a girl-next-door freshness that would compliment her skintones.

◼ The Fast Fabulous Face

If you are in a pinch for time, you can streamline this process by using only five basic products for a fast, fabulous face and doing the following:

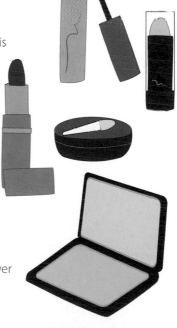

1. **Concealer:** Place under eye area, cover blemishes and smooth out discolorations.

2. **Pressed Powder:** Apply to forehead, nose, chin, and entire eyelid area.

3. **Dark Neutral Shadow:** Contour middle and outer area of eyelid and blend.

4. **Mascara:** Apply one coat on upper and lower lashes.

5. **Lipstick:** Use on lips and also as a cheek color, blend well.

Some people, no matter how old they get never lose their beauty—they merely move it from their faces into their hearts. —Martin Buxbaum

This whole process will take **less than three** minutes and give you that quick "pick me up" as you dash out the door!

◼ Expressions of Beauty

What face do you put on daily for the world? Is it the same one you wear for your family? I read once that a mother's attitude in the morning sets the mood for her family for the rest of their day. What a guilt trip! Like the saying goes, "When Momma ain't happy, ain't nobody happy." My friend Terri adds, "And when Pappa ain't happy, ain't nobody cares." So rather than carry the burden myself, I like to remind my husband, "Happy wife, happy life."

But seriously, while we can't control another's emotions, we do have a choice concerning our attitude. The Bible tells us as Christians we can be mirrors that brightly reflect the glory of the Lord and as the Spirit of the Lord works within us, we become more and more like Him (II Corinthians 3:18 TLB). This means making Jesus *the* top priority in our day. Just as we daily take time to wash our faces and apply moisturizer or makeup, we must also daily take time to pray and apply God's Word to our lives so that it becomes a natural part of our morning ritual.

If you don't have a regular time set aside for Jesus, I encourage you to establish one now. A habit takes twenty-one days to form, so for the next three weeks I challenge you to set up an appointment with God every morning. Start your day thirty minutes earlier than usual. Pour yourself a cup of coffee or tea, find a comfortable chair, and spend some time with the One who cares most about your day. Jesus referred to Himself as the "Bright Morning Star." What a joy to wake up to the risen Son!

You will encounter three blessings when you practice this discipline:

1. The Holy Spirit will help you adjust your attitude.
2. Making daily decisions will become easier.
3. At the end of the day, you will know who to thank as you look back and see prayers answered.

While good and bad days can be subject to circumstances, our attitude doesn't have to be. Smiling and choosing to make the most of any situation with God's help will be a beautiful reflection of His work in our lives.

7 SIMPLE STEPS

1. Clean out the makeup drawer.

2. Toss out any liquid or cream-base products that are over two years old.

3. Scale down your cosmetic collection to three lipsticks, two blushes, and one foundation.

4. Schedule a professional makeup session with a beauty consultant

5. Place your everyday cosmetics in a small basket with easy accessibility.

6. Find a Bible-based devotional book that meets your personal and lifestyle needs.

7. Make a standing appointment to meet with Jesus every morning.

Additional resources:
The Helper by Catherine Marshall
Life Application Bible by Tyndale Publishing

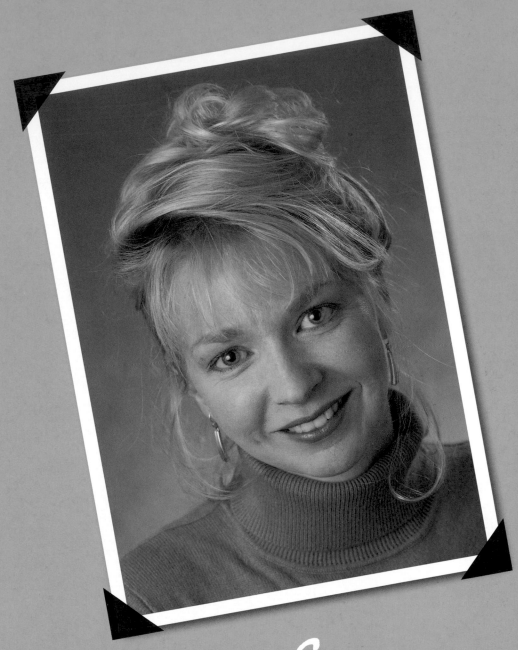

Simply Beautiful

SIGNATURE STYLE

Knowing your personal style is the cornerstone to building a total look that reflects who you really are. Learning to choose clothes with confidence and to feel comfortable when you wear them is the ultimate goal. But how does one determine what her "look" is? The answer is in two small words: *Know thyself.*

God has made you one of a kind, a unique creation needing to express that individuality. Learning how to dress from the inside out will help you feel at ease with your image and add a new dimension of fun and function to your wardrobe.

The Functional Wardrobe

Your lifestyle and personality are important factors in maintaining a functional wardrobe. Lifestyle is defined by where and how you spend your time, and personality determines what criteria to base your choices on. The following exercises will help you evaluate where your closet priorities need to be and how to make successful shopping and every day dressing decisions.

Lifestyle Profile

Take a minute and look at your calendar for the past week. Write down the approximate number of hours you spent at each activity.

___Career/job   ___ Church
___Housework   ___ Volunteer work
___Errands/shopping   ___ Social gatherings
___Exercise/sports   ___ Kids' activities/other

Assign each time slot of activity a letter indicating what you would wear and add up the total for each letter:

Totals:

B ___

C ___

H ___

"B" = Business/dressy clothes (suits, dresses, slacks/jackets, etc…)

"C" = Nice casual clothes (slacks, good jeans, blouses, sweaters, etc…)

"H" = Home/sportswear (t-shirts, shorts, jeans, sweats, etc…)

Now proceed to your closet and evaluate the clothes you own that fall into these three basic areas. How does the amount of time spent in each area compare to the number of clothing items you have for that event/activity? Is there any trace of imbalance? Your wardrobe should reflect the reality of your life and who you are today. Add or subtract pieces to balance out clothing choices that coincide with your current occupation and lifestyle. Make a shopping list of wants and needs and keep it in your purse. Building a wardrobe is a work in progress, and this will help you stay on task.

Personality Dressing

Choosing clothes that suit you physically, emotionally, and mentally begins with your personality. Knowing what to wear will help you feel at ease and confident. This is the key to your personal dress-for-success program, whether you wear suits or sweats. The following test will help you understand what method works best for you in making daily decisions concerning what to wear and how to organize your closet accordingly.

Look at yourself objectively, not as you wish you were, or as you wish you weren't, but how you actually are most of the time. Check the boxes that describe you.

I

- ☐ Like consistency
- ☐ Humble
- ☐ Peacemaker
- ☐ Patient
- ☐ Security-oriented
- ☐ Hesitant
- ☐ Accommodating
- ☐ Reserved
- ☐ Steady
- ☐ Worrier
- ☐ Submissive
- ☐ Tolerant

II

- ☐ Talkative
- ☐ A good promoter
- ☐ Bubbly
- ☐ Optimistic and outgoing
- ☐ Inspiring
- ☐ Like to perform or be on stage
- ☐ A free-spirit
- ☐ Openly expresses emotion
- ☐ Spontaneous
- ☐ Playful
- ☐ A people person
- ☐ Short attention span

III

- ☐ Contemplative, a thinker
- ☐ Planner
- ☐ Set on doing the "right" thing
- ☐ Competent
- ☐ Loyal
- ☐ Loner
- ☐ Cautious
- ☐ Analytical
- ☐ Perfectionist
- ☐ Thoughtful
- ☐ Sensitive
- ☐ Check for accuracy

IV

- ☐ Confident
- ☐ Direct and to the point
- ☐ Persistent
- ☐ Task-oriented
- ☐ Decisive
- ☐ Bottom-line achiever
- ☐ Productive
- ☐ Strong-willed, resistant
- ☐ Ambitious
- ☐ Proud
- ☐ Independent
- ☐ Assertive

Total I _____ *Total II* _____ *Total III* _____ *Total IV* _____

If the majority of your answers fell in one category, read the subsequent comments by that number. If you have equal checks in two categories, read both summaries.

Some of you may have close to the same number of checks in three or perhaps all four groupings, but don't dismay! This simply means that you are a very balanced person and will do best with a variety of options within your wardrobe. The summary for Personality III will likely suit you best.

Personality I

Comfort and ease are the foremost factors in determining what you should wear on a regular basis. You like to keep life at a relaxed and steady pace. Ideally your desire to maintain a low profile works best when you can blend in with the crowd. Dressing up can make you feel as though you are wearing someone else's clothes. Maintaining a wardrobe with a casual air will eliminate that constricted or hemmed-in feeling that you experience when wearing more formal attire.

In your attempts to be comfortable beware of an overly casual look, which can sometimes make you look unkempt or sloppy. Keep your clothing lines simple and stay with sizes that fit you, skimming your bodylines. Invest in decent casual clothes that reflect fine workmanship and quality materials. Take time to put together outfits with accessories that finish the look. Getting your wardrobe in order will help you focus more on others and worry less about yourself, which is the real beauty that others see in you. A kind, servant's heart is a blessing to all.

Personality II

You love to have fun and experience life to the fullest. Therefore, your wardrobe needs to fulfill that criteria. You can confidently break the fashion rules and wear what you feel like wearing despite what others may think or say. Expressing yourself is very important to you whether it's verbal or visual. It is necessary for you to have a wide variety of looks within your closet: some dramatic, others a little romantic, and perhaps a uniform, or even a "costume" that has been toned down to wear for every day.

My dear friend, Sally, is a Personality II. She can wear a darling sailor outfit one day and a peasant blouse with a full skirt and boots the next. It's as though all of life is a stage, and she is one of the stars.

Adjusting your clothes to your mood is the most effective way to make wardrobe decisions. As one who is in tune with her emotions, you know that a wrong choice of clothing can put a damper on your day, while the right one will send your spirit soaring. The biggest downfall you may encounter is boredom with what you own. Rotate things in your closet every three months, storing some of your outfits in a different room where you don't see them. This will keep what you own fresh and will prevent impulsive shopping sprees that can stem from monotony.

Personality III

Your wardrobe confidence is built on looking appropriate for whatever event or role you may play that day. Staying true to yourself and dressing within the parameters of what looks good on you are also high on your list. Since consistency is important, "formula dressing" tends to work best for your overall closet situation. This means creating complete outfits rather than trying to always play the "mix and match" game with a hodgepodge of different pieces.

Concentrate on buying "sets" of clothing, like the brand name groupings that come out at the beginning of a season. Budget for three to five pieces of the ensemble and purchase the matching accessories. While your conservative nature may question the practicality of spending all this money at once, in the end it will prove to be a wise investment. Buying the complete outfit will save you time and money that would be spent trying to perfect the ensemble in an effort to find the best deal. Because your assets lie in being a "detail" person, you will shine when you maintain a personal dress code of being polished and put-together.

Personality IV

You are tuned into the importance of dressing for success. Your natural tendency toward being goal-oriented weaves itself into your closet with clothing that is functional and projects confidence. For your high speed life and wide range of activities, you need clothing that will make the best use of your energy. Keep it simple, with a minimum of details, eliminate things like multiple buttons, fussy accessories that require hourly adjustments, and clothing that constricts movement.

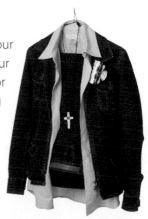

Take time to put three "capsule" outfits together within your closet: (1) a business/professional look, (2) an upscale-casual outfit, and (3) a dressy/glamorous ensemble. Hang everything for each outfit on one hanger, including accessories. This will assist you on days when your schedule is full and time is limited. Knowing the value of outcome-based dressing, your self-assurance will be strongest when you are well dressed for the occasion, and perhaps a notch above the standard. You are in complete control of the way you come across to other people, and you dress accordingly.

Your Outer Image

The third aspect of developing a style that expresses your image, the real you, is found in how you see yourself. Many people have a natural bend towards a look that personifies their fashion identity. For some it is crystal clear and remains consistent throughout their lives. Mary is a perfect example of this. She wears soft colors, prefers dresses to slacks, uses details like ruffles and lace, and loves "Laura Ashley" styles. Mary is a romantic through and through, with a personality that is sweet, gentle, and full of grace. When we first did her style analysis fifteen years ago, she fit the feminine category to a "T." I ran into her recently and observed that she had maintained her romantic look. Charming and approachable as always, she reaffirmed that having her style evaluated and defined was a timeless investment.

Not everyone remains as steady as Mary. Many women tell me they were one style when they were teenagers and have since evolved into a completely different fashion mode. I, for one, went through a romantic phase as a teen, and today only traces of that Victorian look are evident. My natural/classic style has taken over the majority of my wardrobe.

Another factor in our image identity is found in the roles we play. Many times we dress to conform to the event we are placed in, thereby adding an interesting dimension to our wardrobes. Clearly, there are areas of our lives that correspond to specific dressing styles: sportswear for working out, a power suit for business meetings, or a cowboy look for riding horses. We can all use a little variety.

Learning to express yourself from the inside out with a congruent wardrobe is a rewarding experience. Defining your individuality in a personal style that genuinely portrays who you are will help you interact with people and put them at ease. The following test will help you refine your look and make that harmonious connection. Read and follow the directions carefully.

Image Profile

Check the word on each line going <u>across</u> that most describes you or your **preferred** dressing style.

A	B	C	D
☐ Strong	☐ Passionate	☐ Structured	☐ Original
☐ Outdoorsy	☐ Ladylike	☐ Fashionable	☐ Avant-garde
☐ Sporty	☐ Feminine	☐ Timeless	☐ Modern
☐ Physical	☐ Soft	☐ Solid	☐ Abstract
☐ Earthy	☐ Heart-driven	☐ Consistent	☐ Mysterious
☐ Energetic	☐ Gentle	☐ Sophisticated	☐ Contemporary
☐ Green	☐ Pink	☐ Blue	☐ Fuchsia
☐ Wood	☐ Pearls	☐ Polished metals	☐ Artsy
☐ Leather	☐ Lace	☐ Plain	☐ Unique
☐ Suede	☐ Cashmere	☐ Fine wool	☐ Imported fabric
☐ Country style	☐ Victorian style	☐ Business style	☐ Bold style
☐ Plaid	☐ Floral	☐ Stripe	☐ Geometric
☐ Tweed blazer	☐ Soft wrap jacket	☐ Fitted sport coat	☐ Tuxedo jacket
☐ Textured	☐ Flowing	☐ Crisp	☐ Eclectic
☐ Backpack	☐ Soft purse	☐ Structured bag	☐ Trendy tote
☐ Wool jacket	☐ Angora sweater	☐ Chic trench coat	☐ Cape
☐ Earth tones	☐ Pastels	☐ Neutrals	☐ Vivid
Total A's _____	Total B's _____	Total C's _____	Total D's _____

Now that you've tallied up your answers, assess your findings. Were most of your checks clearly in one category? Chances are that your style has already made its mark on your wardrobe. Are there two columns vying for first place? The likely outcome is that you are a "blend" and will be happiest with components of both styles to complete your wardrobe personality.

Undoubtedly, there are those of you who were almost equal in three or four of the groups. No, you are not schizophrenic. A couple of factors could be coming into play. You could be the type of person who prefers a lot of variety, or you may be going through a change in your life that is affecting how you view yourself. A recent move, illness, marital change, and empty-nest syndrome are just a few things that can contribute to how you score on these tests. For example:

Ellen, a woman in her mid-forties, came in for an image consultation recently. After taking several different personality profile tests, her results yielded nothing in terms of a "dominant" style. She later revealed that she was going through a transition phase and was changing careers and reassessing her "life focus." In time, I'm confident that Ellen's look will become more clearly defined as she settles into a new chapter of life.

Another explanation for being equivalent in the categories is that you are a true "versatile classic." The versatile classic woman needs a variety of looks to suit her multi-faceted lifestyle and a wardrobe that is both classic and adaptable. Your fashion will stem from a solid base of traditional, simple styles and draw from the romantic, dramatic, and natural looks by using accessories and unique details to add character to your closet. An example would be dressing up a business suit with a ruffled blouse and pearl earrings to give it a feminine flavor. The same suit can make a dramatic statement by eliminating the blouse, buttoning the jacket, turning up the collar and adding a large scarf over one shoulder. If you feel you are a "versatile," take time to read all four style summaries and pay extra attention to category "C."

Please note that these summaries are meant to give an overview of each look and not to limit your options. As you develop your image identity, you will customize your unique style and, with life experiences, will continue to explore new ones.

Image Profile Summaries

Column A – The Natural

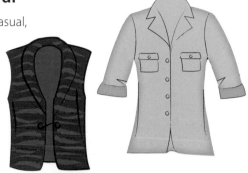

Naturals can range from being earthy and casual, to sporty and energetic. Dressing for comfort and utility is top priority. With a down-to-earth style and a "girl-next-door" freshness, the look is comfortable and current. Separates should make up the bulk of this wardrobe with an emphasis on textured fabrics and handcrafted or artist inspired accessories. The goal is to mix function with fashion to suit an active lifestyle.

Fabrics: Choose a variety of textures and weights to add that unique casual feel to your look. Try cotton, raw silk, flannel, tweed, gauze, camel hair, suede, nubby finishes, sand-washed silk, denim, and corduroy.

Prints: Check, plaid, animal, tapestry, Indian, jungle, unique floral, nature inspired, abstract, and woven.

Accessories: Textured scarves, wearable art, reptile, wood, woven leather, tortoise shell, hammered metals, natural beads and natural pearls, chains, rope belts, and anything that suggests a bit of nature.

Details: Leather piping, suede patches, braids, epaulets, fringe, safari, heavy embroidery, western, military looks, jumpsuits, and bib overalls.

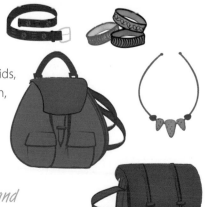

Famous Naturals:
Meg Ryan, Amy Grant, Carol Burnett, and
Christie Brinkley

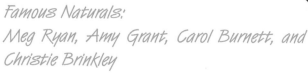

Column B – The Romantic

The Romantic is the epitome of ageless beauty. The look can be interpreted as feminine, delicate, elegant, or glamorous, but the heart of this style is *softness.* Choose flowing silhouettes that subtly show the curves of your body, waist definition, or gentle draping with fluid fabrics. Whether it's lavish details or none at all, the essence of a romantic can be seen in the soft lines and the special touches that make this individual approachable and irresistible.

Fabrics: Chiffon, crepe, thin cotton, silk, velvet, tissue linen, cashmere, angora, rayon, lace, fine wool flannel, brushed denim, no-wale cord, sheer wool, and delicate crochet knits.

Prints: Soft solids, thin stripes, floral patterns, lace overlay, watercolor, tone-on-tone effects, antique looks, and cascading flowers.

Accessories: Pearls, lockets, cameos, silk flowers, lace scarves, camisoles, feathers, butter-soft leather, sashes, ribbons, chiffon scarves, soft brimmed hats, delicate shoes, and purses with ovalized lines.

Details: Rounded edges, soft to the touch, ruffles, lace, soft embroidery, bows, pearl buttons, eyelet, puffed sleeves, delicate embossing, and draped looks.

Famous Romantics:
Meryl Streep, Dolly Parton, Liz Taylor,
and Ce Ce Winans

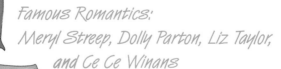

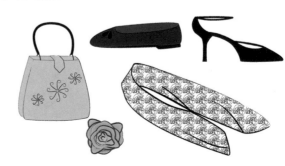

Column C – The Classic

The Classic has a look that is polished, timeless, and elegant. The hallmarks of a classic wardrobe are simplicity and refined style. Like the eternal diamond that never loses its luster or value, the longevity of this collection is rooted in quality workmanship and traditional pieces. Clothing with smooth lines that are tailored to skim the body and minimal details showcase the Classic's distinguished taste. A coordinated look from head-to-toe is essential in creating a balanced look.

Fabrics: High quality should be top priority. Try: wool challis, silk, crisp cotton, broadcloth, jersey, linen, ultra suede, fine wool, cashmere, crepe, calf, or kidskin leather.

Prints: Smooth solids, evenly spaced designs, plaids, stripes, pinstripe, herringbone, houndstooth, subtle geometrics, paisley, and marble effects.

Accessories: One important piece per outfit. Matched sets of jewelry, slightly geometric shapes, sculpted smooth designs, silk scarves, fine leather goods, dress boots, fedora hat, and quality belts.

Details: Well-cut garments, fitted looks, understated, simple, unadorned, smooth silhouettes, coordinated, expensive look

Famous Classics:
Grace Kelly, Connie Chung, Anne Graham
Lotz, and Nancy Reagan

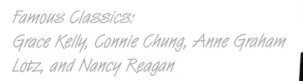
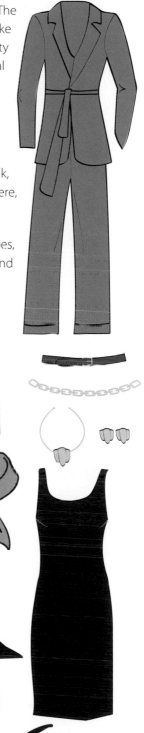

Column D – The Dramatic

Distinguished by daring styles and unpredictable fashion statements, the Dramatic's independent attitude sets the tone for this bold look. Contemporary, eclectic, and exotic are just a few words that describe this individualized style that commands attention. Experiment with innovative ways of wearing ordinary clothing and accessorize with unique signature pieces. Shun the latest trends and integrate "one-of-a-kind" designs to create a wardrobe that is ultra chic.

Fabrics: Tightly woven or smooth surfaces, leather, jersey wool, crepe, muslin, wool challis, velvet, brocade, silk, stretch cotton, sequins, satin, raw silk, and metallic knits.

Prints: Bold geometrics, strong solids, dramatic florals, asymmetric, zig zag, abstracts, contemporary, exotic, and high contrast.

Accessories: Demanding pieces, sculptured looks, fun shoes, unique glasses, European style, boots, gloves, hats, large scarves, and wild purses.

Details: Minimal, modern, artsy, unusual, angular shapes, asymmetrical, ethnic, and sharp edges.

Famous Dramatics:
Ann Coutier, Della Reese,
Kathy Trocolli and Nicole C. Mullen

Hairs the Deal

Your hairstyle is the unspoken theme of your appearance. It reflects your lifestyle and gives insight into your personality. It often echoes your mood, and it definitely affects it. A bad hair day can deflate self-esteem. I have seen a fuzzy perm reduce our most stoic sister to tears. While a ponytail makes us feel young, a French twist gives a sophisticated air. We can all relate to the four stages of hair – too long, too short, too straight, and too curly. Finding our ideal hairstyle seems to be the proverbial "pot of gold" at the end of the elusive rainbow.

The following are some simple suggestions to ease the stresses of the tresses.

Assess What You Have

Is it up to date? Many women live in a time warp with their hair. Do any of the following describe your look? Cher and the long straight hair of the 60's, Barbara Streisand's poodle top and Farrah Fawcett's mane of the 70's, and the voluptuous styles of the evening soap operas, such as Dynasty and Falcon Crest, in the 80's? The 90's ushered in a messy Meg Ryan look and the still-popular Jennifer Aniston modified shag. What you were complimented on ten or twenty years ago may not be consistent with what looks good on you now. As faces and bodies change over the decades, we need to adjust our hairstyle to enhance our features and not detract from them.

Does your hair look good most of the time? If you can't do the do, it's time to try something new. A hairstyle must be conducive to your daily routine and your ability to achieve it. By the same token, don't make a hasty decision to cut it when you are having a bad hair day. Are you consistently feeling it makes you look "frumpy" or old? Then that is your indicator to try a new style.

Is it really you? Your hairstyle should reflect your own personal style. For example: if you have a "classic" style, your hair should be tailored and well cut. If you are a "natural," something easy like a ponytail or casual messy look is good. Perhaps you are more fashion forward, dramatic, and trendy. Try a cutting edge style to suit your individuality as well as your wardrobe. Romantics will want softness and many times some curl. A soft updo with gentle tendrils framing the face is the quintessential feminine trait.

Find a Stylist

Ask around! If you see someone whose hair you admire and it appears to have a similar texture to your own (fine, curly, etc.), take a minute to inquire as to who her stylist is. Most women are flattered to have someone take notice.

In the event that you are ready to make a major change in your hairstyle, pay the extra money and use the top stylist in the salon. It is worth it since that person has had extra training and experience. If you like the style, often times you can book with a rookie in the same salon, and the master stylist will guide that hairdresser in the cutting and styling techniques used.

Seek out hair designers who have a gift for cutting, styling, and/or coloring hair. Some are naturally talented in these areas and will do the best work.

Take advantage of the free consultations offered at salons. This will help guide you in what would look good on you as well as establish a relationship with the stylist. If you don't feel comfortable with the person, or her advice, you can move elsewhere without a risk.

Choose the Right Style

Consider your face, body shape, and features. Seek to achieve balance between the volume of hair and the size and height of your body. For example: larger body = fuller hair. Petite body = chic hair. An attractive hairstyle is all about balance. It should be proportioned to the width of your shoulders and your height, as well as the unique details of your face and its shape. Here are some tips to help you find a suitable style:

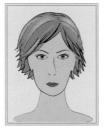

Oblong/rectangular face does well with soft bangs to add fullness at the forehead. A side or asymmetrical part works best.

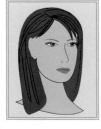 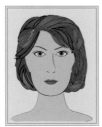

Round/wide face is complemented by styles with a diagonal line, an off-center part, or a bang that lifts in one spot at the roots. A fringe bang, where you can see parts of the forehead is also good.

A short, square or round face is flattered most with some height at the front of the crown or top of head.

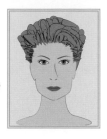

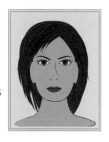

Pear shape/broad jaw line needs soft curls or fullness across the forehead to balance with lower half of face.

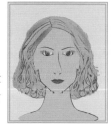

Heart shape/wide forehead benefits from a style that adds volume at the chin level with a slightly off-center part.

The shorter your forehead is, the longer your bangs should be.

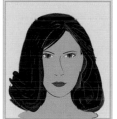

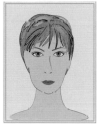

Proportion your hair to your face size. A large face needs a fuller hairstyle, and a smaller head looks better with less volume.

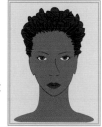

A short, curly haircut can give you more height if it is cut narrow at the sides.

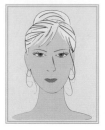

Wearing long hair up will make your neck look longer and your body look slimmer (so will most short styles).

Ultimately, the perfect hairstyle communicates our personality, enhances our face and features, and suits our lifestyle.

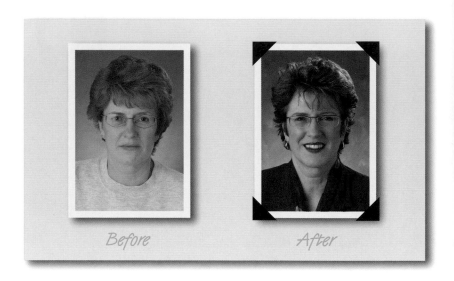

Before   *After*

A warmer hair color and perky style that lifts the bangs off the forehead, brightens Terri's face and brings her beautiful features into balance.

Hair Products to Simplify Your Life

Hair accessories that match your hair color. When the barrette or band blends, it will coordinate with whatever you are wearing. This would include: rubber bands, ponytail holders, hair combs, clips, and headbands. If you can't find a similar color, try spray-painting them yourself. I've done this, and it works great.

Cheap shampoo, such as Suave or generic brands, can double as liquid soap in your shower and works especially well from a pump style bottle.

Hairpieces. The key here is to get a color that matches perfectly to your hair and a texture that looks natural. The elasticized curly bun works well for almost anyone, especially that person with short hair who wants to wear her hair pulled back in a pony-tail, but it isn't quite long enough. The braided add-ons also work well and give some variety to your look.

Instant-heat curlers. Hot rollers and curling irons are now designed to heat within a 1-2 minute period, saving precious time in the hairstyling process. Choose irons and curling sets with "velvet" flocking on the rods (to prevent hair from slipping out when you are trying to roll it). A set of large "butterfly clips" will hold hot curlers in place and make the job much quicker and easier.

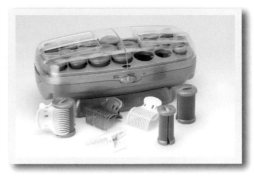

Maintenance

Before committing to a new style, ask how difficult or easy it is to maintain. A good stylist is willing to teach you the techniques necessary to do it. If you can't or don't want to bother with it, choose a different cut.

If your bangs need a little trim, and you want to save some time, try cutting them yourself using pinking shears. I also suggest you do it when they are dry to avoid "shrinkage."

Blow-dry your hair upside down to give it extra volume and lift.

If you have medium to long hair and do not want to wash it the next day, wear it in a ponytail on the top of your head when you go to sleep. Use soft, thick, fabric-covered elastic. To help hair retain its curl, you can form the tail into a bun, mushroom style, and secure it with bobby pins. The next morning when you take it down, you can just brush, fluff, and go.

Make peace with the texture and type of mane you've been blessed with, or to put it another way: *Be content with such hair that you have, for someday it may leave you or forsake you!*

Interior Designing

Fashion is fun! Letting go and expressing ourselves through the clothes we wear gives us the opportunity to reflect different facets of our personality and enjoy the individuality God created in each one of us. For some, fashion is an avenue to exhibit creativity or a means of non-verbal communication; for others it's all about comfort. Regardless of how we use it, the clothing, hairstyles, and accessories we select shape the image we project to the rest of the world.

Though we consider exterior decorating important, we must place the greatest emphasis on that which leaves the most lasting impression—the interior decorating. Dr. Elizabeth Kubler-Ross once said, "People are like stained-glass windows. They sparkle and shine when the sun is out, but when the darkness sets in, their true beauty is revealed only if there is a light from within."

This reminds me of some houses I saw at a TV studio in Hollywood. The exteriors were beautiful with perfectly groomed lawns, newly painted shutters, and not a shingle out of place. However, on the inside they were hollow, empty shells—a façade to make you believe there was life and beauty inside.

For some of us do-it-yourselfers, redecorating is just a motivational book away. We fool ourselves into thinking we can accomplish the task as easily as taking a course or implementing a behavioral modification program. When we attempt these projects without God's help, they prove to be nothing more than fancy window treatments that look good only from the outside, but eventually fade and deteriorate with time. For lasting results, we need to contact the Master Designer who holds the original blueprints to our life's plan.

I'll never forget the day I called on God to take over my own remodeling job. I started this renovation when I was young, feeling confident that with the right skills and perseverance I could run my own life. After years of trying, the task became monumental. The foundation of pride that I built on was beginning to crumble. Sin had found a home in my heart, and my life was in a shambles.

I fell to my knees that warm spring afternoon and tearfully handed the keys to Jesus. After confessing and apologizing for the mess I had made, I inquired about the price. He told me it was paid in full. With mercy and love He forgave me and transformed my life. He introduced me to His Holy Spirit who now dwells within me as the keeper of my soul, illuminating me from the inside out with real joy.

If you are interested in contracting out your interior decorating project to God, I would highly recommend it. He loves you and wants to help. He can be reached through a simple prayer like this one:

Lord, I need you. I'm sorry for the things I've done wrong in my life, please forgive me. I believe you sacrificed yourself to pay for the things I've done wrong so I can have a relationship with you. Be my Savior, and help me live my life for you. I want to experience the joy that comes from walking in obedience with you and the presence of your Holy Spirit. Thank you, Lord. In Jesus' name, Amen.

The Bible says:

For it is by grace you have been saved, through faith—and this not from yourselves, it is the gift of God. (Ephesians 2:8)

Enjoy this gift and let God do the decorating.

7 SIMPLE STEPS

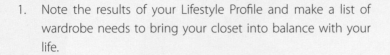

1. Note the results of your Lifestyle Profile and make a list of wardrobe needs to bring your closet into balance with your life.

2. Review your Personality Profile(s) and write out three words that will help you focus on choosing your everyday clothes.

    _____

    _____

    _____

3. Make a collage that reflects your image type by going through clothing catalogs or fashion magazines and tearing out pictures of your style: natural, romantic, dramatic, or classic.

4. Do an accessory search in your closet for pieces that already mirror your style.

5. Assess your current hairstyle and determine what changes you need to make.

6. Are you in need of any "interior decorating?" Read the book of John in your Bible. Then ask God to help you remodel areas that may require attention.

7. If you prayed the prayer at the end of this chapter, make a commitment to read God's Word, pray, and join a Bible-based church to help you learn to grow spiritually in your walk with Jesus.

Additional resources:
Your Spiritual Personality by Marita Littauer
Personality Plus: How to Understand Others by Understanding Yourself
    by Florence Littauer

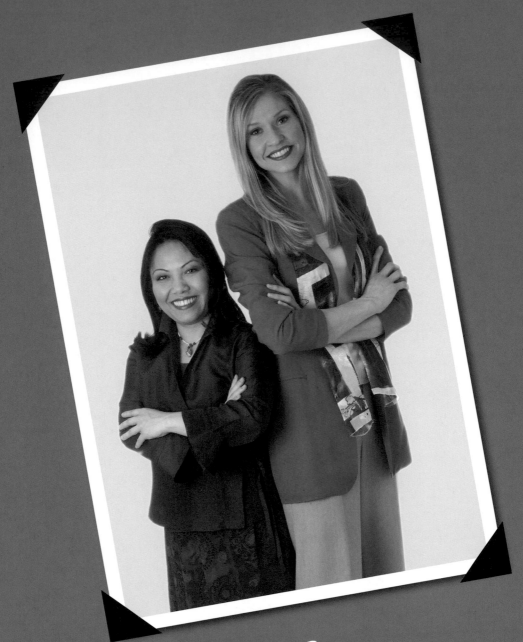

Simply Beautiful

FACTS AND FIGURES 5

Nothing is beautiful from every point of view.
—Quintus Horatius Flaccus Horace,
18th Century Roman poet

Too often, as women, we tend to desire the "ideal body," forever obsessing over the "imperfections" our own critical eye sees in the mirror. By measuring ourselves against unrealistic pictures of beautiful women in magazines and on TV we corrupt our self-image and move dangerously close to idolatry, putting too much time and energy into trying to become something we envy.

No body is perfect, so let's just get over ourselves and come to terms with where we are physically. To get comfortable with the body we've been blessed with, we need to assess what we have, accent the positives, and eliminate the negatives. Balancing our build through the fit and design of our clothing choices does this. As my missionary friend, Melissa, used to say: "Clothes cover a multitude of sins." I couldn't agree more.

Universal Style Tips

There are styles and dressing techniques with universal flattering power that every woman should be aware of. The following is a list of tips to help you make the most of what you've got.

In 1972, twenty-three percent of American women were dissatisfied with their appearance; by 1997 that figure had risen to fifty-six percent.

Ten Tips to Lose Ten Pounds Instantly

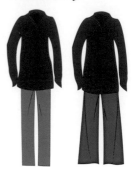

1. Never wear two tight fitting pieces together or two loose pieces together. Pair a fitted piece with a loose piece: Flowing soft top with fitted pants or fitted top with a fuller bottom.

Pleats add pounds

2. Create one area of interest in an outfit, either near the face or at the most flattering part of the body. Too many accent colors or accessories tend to make one look like a dispersed puzzle.

3. Unless you are going out for the Olympic gymnastic team or a ballet troupe, save the spandex and tight clingy clothes for your aerobics class.

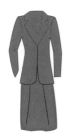

4. Separates are most flattering when one top piece is the same or a similar color as the bottom (i.e. shirt and skirt matching or jacket and slacks) with an open line running vertically without interruption. Add a bright or unique color on the upper half of the body such as a scarf or contrasting jacket worn open.

5. Shoulder pads are your friends. Choose those that add width by rounding over the edge of the shoulder. They should blend with the garment style and be completely unnoticeable. Remove or reduce shoulder pads when necessary.

6. Keep clothing simple in your "weighty" areas. Whether it's the thighs, stomach, hips, or bust, the less detailed and more streamlined, the better.

7. Recognize that bulky fabrics add bulk: hand-knits, tweed, and wide corduroy are all like wearing double the material. Choose thin fabrics such as silk, crepe, light cottons, or tropical weight wool.

8. Work at eliminating "line breaks." Any horizontal line will cut an inch of length off in the area it's worn, whether it is a ruffle, cuff, or contrasting trim. Wearing the same or monochromatic colors in an area minimizes horizontal lines that are created by color differences.

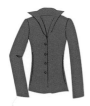

9. To look taller, thinner, and frame your face in a flattering way turn the back of your collar up halfway, "Elvis style."

10. Sit up straight.

■ Creating HAVOX

Now we get down to the nitty-gritty of dealing with individual body types. It's time to intimately acquaint yourself with the body you have today. Take a deep breath and put on a solid color one-piece swimsuit or leotard. Begin by standing in front of a full-length mirror. Pretend you are looking at a stranger. Analyze the overall silhouette of the body. Are you small on the top and large on the bottom or the other way around? Do you have a "round" shape or are you more straight up and down? I have found that most women fall into one of five designs: H, A, V, O, or X.

Note: If it is difficult for you to assess your own physique, have someone take pictures of you (front, side and rear views with a solid contrasting background). This is the easiest and most accurate way to study your own body objectively.

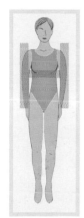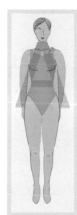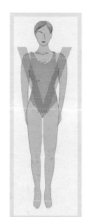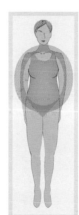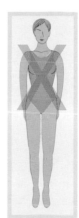

The **"H"** body is generally short-waisted and long-legged, without a "definable" waistline. She can be thin or have a broader build but is straight up-and-down.

The **"A"** body, often called the "pear-shape" has a small upper torso and a fuller thigh and buttock area.

The **"V"** body is broad through the shoulders/bust area with a narrow hip line.

The **"O"** body is a voluptuous woman with a fuller figure.

The **"X"** body is an hourglass shape with bust and hips in proportion to each other and waist visually smaller.

Distinct Differences

Before I launch into giving you all sorts of figure flattering tips, I need to insert a disclaimer. Different body types have different challenges. Not everybody is going to benefit from all the tips in their respective categories. In my years of working with thousands of different shapes and sizes, I've discovered that there are no absolutes—God created each body unique!

Dressing to the Letter
"H"

Goal: Create the illusion of having curves in your shape by adding width or interest at the shoulder and hip areas and elongating the waist.

TRY	AVOID
Moderate shoulder pads	Wide waistbands or belts
No-waist dresses	High-cut slacks
Shirts/sweaters over slacks	Horizontal lines/details on torso
Skirts/slacks with no waistband	Contrasting colors at the waistline
Single color outfits with interest near the face or leg area (i.e. knee-length jacket with slacks)	Pleated pants
Vertical and long diagonal lines on upper half of body	Cropped shirts and sweaters
A bra that lifts the bust-line up to give a longer waist look	
Petite sizes for dresses and shirts	

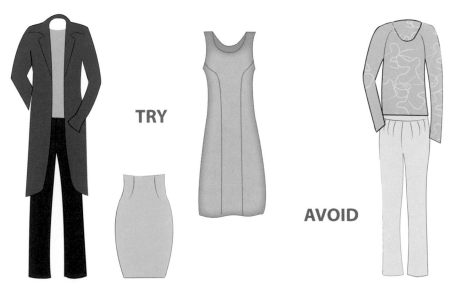

TRY

AVOID

"A"

Goal: To elongate the legs, showcase the waist, and broaden the shoulder/bust area giving balance to the wide hip area.

TRY	AVOID
Single button blazers	Cuffs on slacks/shorts
Shoulder pads/broad shoulder lines	Pleats/gathers at waist
Clothes that skim the body below the waist	Hip huggers
Belts same color as pant/skirt	Styles without waist definition
Perfect fit pants	Jackets that end at fullest part of hip
Sew slit pockets shut on skirts and slacks and remove lining	Capri or crop-style pants
Hose, shoes, slacks/skirt matched	Spandex or tight fabric below waist
Straight-leg or slightly flared pants	
Padded bra	
Trouser leg falls over shoe	

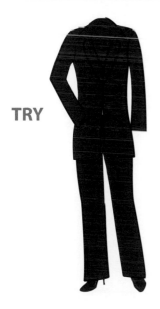

TRY

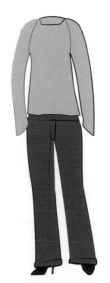

AVOID

"V"

Goal: Lengthen the waist area and show off the legs.

TRY	AVOID
No waist band on skirts/slacks	Horizontal detail from the waist up
Drop waist styles and low-slung belts	Short jackets and vests
Slim shirts and sweaters worn over skirts and slacks	Bulky sweaters and tops
Hip huggers and low hung pants	Wide belts and waistbands
Soft fabrics and simple lines on top	Boxy style tops and jackets
Belts that match tops	Large shoulder pads
Flared skirts	Double-breasted jackets
Open necklines	
Long over-blouses and jackets	
A minimizer bra	

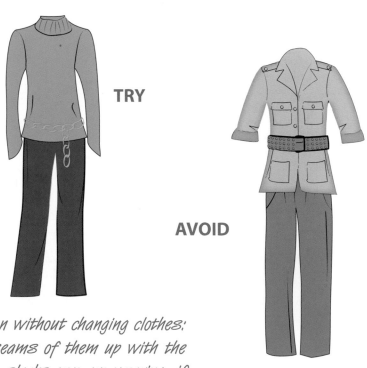

TRY

AVOID

To try pants on without changing clothes: line the side seams of them up with the seams on the slacks you are wearing, if they don't match, don't bother with them.

"O"

Goal: Wear clothing that gently drapes from the shoulders, skimming the body and complementing the face.

TRY	AVOID
Curved shoulder pads that broaden the shoulders	Sloping shoulder lines
Slightly flared skirts	Belts and waist detail
Monochromatic or single colored outfits	Anything too small
Long straight-cut tops that skim the body	Cropped or short pants
Slightly long slacks	Short jackets or vests
No waist dresses with strong shoulder lines	Gathers visible at waist
Unstructured and soft fluid designs	Tucked in shirts
Unbroken lines from top to bottom	
Long diagonal or vertical details	

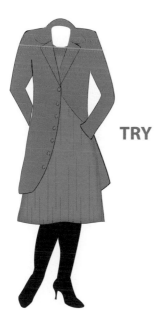

TRY

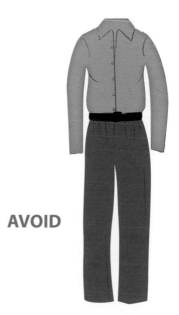

AVOID

Goal: To keep the figure balanced and trim-looking overall.

TRY	AVOID
Keep clothing lines smooth and symmetrical	Too many details
Diagonal lines	Clothes that do not fit properly
Knee-length skirts	

This list is short. Bear in mind that you have been blessed with the "ideal" physique; the need to adjust and balance your body is minimal.

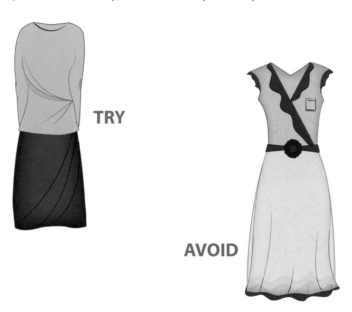

TRY

AVOID

■ **Fashionably Fit**

Giving the illusion of a more perfect body is an art that can be mastered. We see it done in Hollywood, magazine spreads and mail order catalogs. Often it leaves the rest of us yearning for liposuction and personal trainers. The truth is the fashion model's body actually has little to do with the result. Aside from some airbrushing and technological wizardry, there is another secret to looking great in those clothes that the average woman can implement. It's as close as your nearest needle and thread: alterations. Getting the proper fit to clothing can compliment your body, making you look slimmer and well dressed.

A beautiful woman lacking discretion and modesty is like a fine gold ring in a pig's snout. Prov. 11:22 TLB

Here's the reality:

1. Clothes that are too big make you look heavy.

2. Clothes that are too small make you look fat.

3. Clothes that fit you perfectly will make you look like a million dollars.

The problem comes from the fact that most of us don't understand what a well-fitted garment looks like.

Women's clothing retailers would have us believe that all of us are built with an average body shape and fit into the standard sizes they sell: 8, 10, 12 etc. Yet, when a man buys a suit, and tries it on, there magically appears "The Great Mendini," a tailor who fits it to his physique and gives his body the illusion of perfection. When was the last time you had that happen in the ladies suit department? Give us a break. We women have a lot more bumps and curves than our male counterparts.

We need to develop a keen eye for what fits and what doesn't. Here is a list of subtle indicators that will help you achieve this.

A garment does NOT fit if:

*   **You can grab a handful of fabric** from the back of your buttoned suit jacket or fitted dress.

*   **Pleats and darts don't lay flat.** Puckered pants add two or more inches to your stomach and hips.

*   **Garments pull or tug on you anywhere.** Your clothes should allow you to move freely.

*   **There are strained buttons or closures.**

*   **Slacks have a droopy seat or crotch.** Test this by rolling the waistband one turn; if the fit looks better try a smaller size or different style.

*   **Clothes crease or gap horizontally.** This is an indication that the garment is too small.

- **Clothes don't move when they should.** Sleeves that glue to your arms when you stretch forward or pants that don't slide up when you sit make you uncomfortable throughout the day.

- **Clothes shift when they shouldn't.** Collars and shoulders that drop toward the back or jeans that need to be constantly re-adjusted for comfort are a hassle we can do without.

- **Outlines of undergarments are visible.** Those unsightly V.P.L.'s (Visible Panty Lines) can prove to be an advertisement for underwear or a focal point for pants that are too tight.

- **The waistband is tight or gaping.** You should be able to put two fingers under the waistband comfortably, no more and no less.

- **Clothes cling like your skin.** Whether it shows the dimples in the thighs, the banana rolls on the abdomen, or the round curve of your buttocks, they don't do anyone over the age of ten justice. Fitted clothing should gently hug the body, not strangle it.

One final word for us hopeless dieters:

- **Have one "fat day" outfit that looks great on you and is comfortable.** It will be worth its weight in gold.

Clothing can make a powerful statement but, choosing the right fit and style for our body can give us a polished look and take ten pounds off without diet or exercise!

▆ Every Body Is Unique

A heart at peace gives life to the body.
Proverbs 14:30a

There are several things I'd like to change about my body: longer legs, smaller feet, and a more balanced bust to hip ratio for starters. At 5'3", a size nine shoe and a derriere proportionately larger than my chest, I resemble a duck. These are some of the quirks I've had to learn to live with. As I ponder my imperfect components, I'm aware of how God has used these deficiencies to shape my character and forge my spiritual growth. But there is one part of my anatomy that I would not change although many would say it is my most unattractive feature. Looking down at my bare midriff, rather than being a smooth, sleek abdomen, like the ones exposed in the media and on the streets, mine resembles a street map in and of itself.

Since birth, I've had nine surgeries to correct an intestinal malformation called gastroschisis. Doctors have rearranged and removed things in an effort to relieve the chronic pain that mounts and coincides with the obstructions caused by a birth defect. Going in for a tune up about every five years or 50,000 miles, whichever comes first, is routine maintenance for me; but I'm no martyr by any means, and the E.R. personnel will confirm that. One doctor said she had never heard someone scream so loudly. Since having my large intestine removed, I'm sure I will always be remembered as the "gutless wonder" that I am today.

With each new scar comes healing, revelation, and spiritual maturity. Many who have been through physical and medical battles with Jesus next to them will confirm that it is no picnic, but it can be a blessing. The things we learn through the trials of life are jewels that make us shine brighter and exude the light of the Spirit within us. Whether we're laid aside by illness or called aside for stillness—how we respond will depend on who's holding our hand.

God created your body just for you. Learn to accept what you've been blessed with and remember to:

…Be content with what you have, because God has said, *"Never will I leave you; never will I forsake you." (Hebrews 13:5b)*

7 SIMPLE STEPS

1. Do your own body analysis. Put on a leotard and size yourself up in a full-length mirror and determine if you are an H, A, V, O, or X.

2. Review the clothes you have in your closet and assess what they do for your assets and where they create liabilities.

3. Purge your closet of clothing that does not fit you correctly and have it altered or give it away.

4. Make note of the brand and sizes that do fit you well for future shopping references.

5. Choose the hem length that flatters your leg the most. Try one just below the kneecap where the calf begins to curve in at the back of the leg.

6. Invest in one "Fat Day" outfit.

7. Make peace with the body you've been blessed with; God formed it with you in mind and the purpose He has for you on this earth.

Additional resources:
Joni by Joe Musser

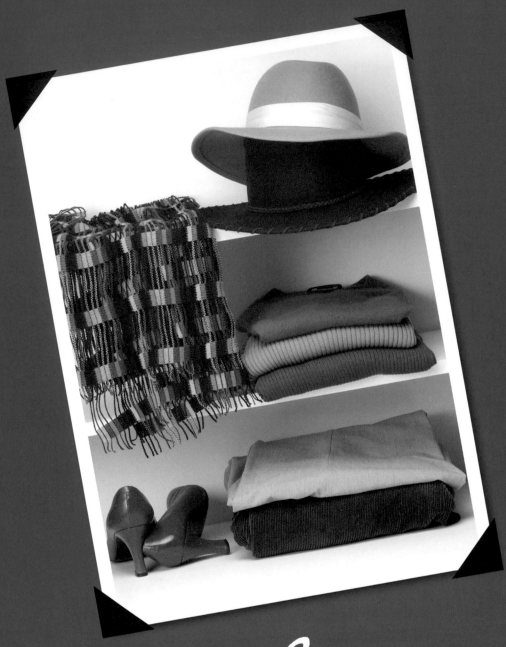

Simply Beautiful

DOWNSIZING THE CLOSET

The average woman wears about ten percent of the clothes in her closet ninety percent of the time. Sound familiar? After seeing hundreds of closets in my line of work, I can verify that statistic. We have our favorite outfits we wear again and again, and a multitude of "other" clothes we wear out of guilt or obligation. I think it all started with Eve, just after the fall. She got up early one morning, surveyed her wardrobe and exclaimed, "I've got a closet full of fig leaves and nothing to wear!"

Whether it's fig leaves or clothes, many of us have closets that resemble a natural disaster. Some of us continuously add pieces without regard to creating outfits while others develop time capsules, stockpiling garments as the decades roll by.

I recently sorted a closet for a woman whose life was undergoing a major transition. After twenty-three years of living in the same house, raising her family, and being active in the community, her husband's company was transferring them to the East Coast. Lesley was determined to condense her closet before the move. She gave me a tour of three bulging closets, nine overstuffed dresser drawers and a loaded antique cedar chest. As we pulled her clothes out, one piece at a time, each revealed a chapter in her life. Lesley's collection amassed a rich history of memories, along with a wardrobe that had long expired without a proper burial. The artifacts included the tight fit, the misfit, and the unfit, as well as numerous things that no longer worked with her current lifestyle. It was time to start letting go. She bravely watched as the "tired and expired" pile grew taller.

A popular song reminds us that "breaking up is hard to do," and where there's emotional attachment to clothing, I know that it's true. Once Lesley survived the "tough love" wardrobe session, she was ready to move on to her new life. A month later I received a note from her, saying that organizing and purging her closet was the best thing she ever did for herself. She felt confident about her appearance and free at last from the burden of clutter.

Now it's your turn. If you are serious about simplifying your wardrobe, there is no better place to start than decluttering the closet and no better time than now. The very thought of this can be overwhelming for some. Stop here, take a deep breath, and imagine the long-term benefits. Through this experience you will:

- Discover "new" outfits hidden among your old pieces

- Save time and frustration when you open your closet

- Look put together and feel more confident

- Realize that less is more and a lot easier to take care of

Prepare to embark on an exciting and rewarding adventure as you journey to the depths of your closet.

■ READY, GET SET, GO!

Step 1: Have a Plan

What is your goal? Is it to simply tidy up or to revamp your entire wardrobe? At some point in time, "tidying up" will not rectify the problem, and eventually clothes will be bulging out of your closet and drawers. It's time to get real.

When are you going to do it? Set a date on your calendar. To accomplish your goal, a full day and an empty house are vital. Choose a day when the rest of the family is gone. Hire a sitter outside of your home, or swap time with a friend for childcare.

Who is going to do it? If you are the type of person who has a hard time letting go of things, you will need help. Choose an *honest* friend or relative whose style you admire and who will be *ruthless*. You need someone who will tell you if an outfit makes you look ten pounds heavier or like you just stepped off the circus train.

Step 2: Get Set

The following is a list of supplies that will help you in this endeavor.

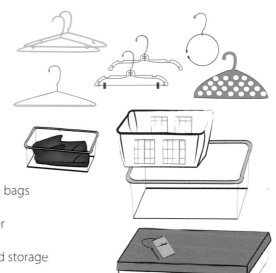

- ☐ Plastic or wooden hangers

- ☐ Single pants hangers

- ☐ Suit hangers with skirt clips

- ☐ Clothes basket

- ☐ Full length mirror

- ☐ Large box or heavy duty garbage bags

- ☐ Trunk or plastic covered container

- ☐ Large flat boxes for under the bed storage

- ☐ Small notebook with pen attached

Assess your current closet situation. Do you need to better utilize the space above or below the hanging clothes? This is a good time to consider adding more shelves or having closet rods double hung. For most, only a small amount of space is needed for longer hanging clothes like dresses. Discount and hardware stores carry simple wire grids and shelves that are easy to install. Keep shelves shallow in depth; 12-15 inches is best. Another option would be to redo the entire space with a "closet insert." This is a clever shelving system that can be tailored to meet your needs and is available at most major hardware stores.

Go through the household organizing department of a discount or hardware store and take time to look over other products that would be beneficial to your closet. For example, you may want to consider: a belt holder, scarf organizer, a hanging jewelry bag, clear shoe boxes, and shoe racks.

Don't buy spontaneously. Only get the things you know you will use. Once you've finished the job, you may discover other organizing items that will suit your needs. In the meantime, here is what *not* to buy:

- Tiered pant/skirt hangers are inconvenient to use, and you can't see at a glance what you have hanging on them.

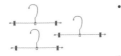

- Skirt hangers tend to "lock" into each other. Hang skirts on suit hangers.

- "Organizers" can cause the garment or accessory to be hidden from view. Out of sight, out of mind; if you don't see it, you won't use it.

- Containers or gadgets that take more than one simple motion to access (i.e. belt holders where you have to remove five belts to get to the one you want).

Clothes need room to breathe and air-out between wearings, therefore, eliminate all metal hangers from your closet (with the exception of the pant hangers with the cardboard tube). Use wood or plastic hangers like you would find in a clothing store. These will make your closet more user-friendly and you won't be fighting with hangers to get the clothes out. If you choose the plastic tube type hanger, buy heavy duty ones and only in white or light color; the darker colors have been known to fade onto fabrics.

When doing this job alone, a camcorder is useful. Set the camera on a table at one end of the room, then video yourself in each outfit front and back. You can be your own critic, and this will give you an accurate assessment of how well each piece fits, whether it is flattering, and if the color works for you.

I video taped my own outfits, and I had so much fun going through my basic wardrobe I decided to do my lingerie. It was a hoot! I viewed the tape, rewound it, and learned some valuable lessons. The main one: when you finish the project, destroy the evidence. A month later, I hosted a bridal shower for a friend. Her mom forgot to bring a video tape and asked to borrow one of mine. The following week she called to tell me that her dad said, "I really enjoyed the video of your shower; especially the fashion show at the end." I was so embarrassed!

Step 3: Go for It!

When the day comes, prepare yourself mentally, physically, and spiritually:

1. Say a prayer, and let I Chronicles 28:20 motivate you:

    "Be strong and courageous and get to work. Don't be frightened by the size of the task, for the Lord my God is with you; He will not forsake you. He will see to it that everything is finished correctly." (TLB)

2. Dress in easy-to-change clothes. Put on a little makeup and do your hair. Looking good is essential in making an accurate evaluation.

3. Open the shades to allow as much natural light as possible into the room and/or turn on all the lights. Add extra temporary lighting if necessary.

4. Make the bed and clear out all the room clutter. You will need all the space you can find.

5. Set your mirror up at one end of the room for an unobstructed view. Have all of your supplies on hand.

6. Bring in your accomplice or set the video camera up and adjust the height and distance so that you can view yourself from head to toe.

■ FINDERS, KEEPERS...

Make a game out of this project and have some fun! Take each piece of clothing out of the closet and try it on, coordinating an outfit. Model it for your friend and in front of the mirror. If you are using the video method, turn the camera on and strut your stuff, front and back. Turn it off between ensembles. Listen to your friend and your gut instinct. As you evaluate each piece, ask:

Do I like it?

Do I need it?

Do I wear it? (...Not "Will I wear it!")

Then move on to *divide and conquer*. The easiest way to go about this project is to put each piece of clothing into one of the following categories:

Finders,

Keepers,

Losers,

Weepers.

■ Finders

Every woman has perfectly good clothes in her closet that hang dormant month after month because she must *find* something in order to make them wearable. We use excuses like:

"If I could *find* the right shirt to go with this, I would wear it."

"If I could *find* the time to hem this, I would use it."

"If I could *find* a way to lose ten pounds, I'd fit into this."

These are the dark clouds that hang in our closets. They remind us of all the things we have to do or don't want to do. If it is a matter of gaining or losing weight, set a date on the calendar (within the next six months) to alter your body to that size. If you don't attain your goal by then, get rid of the clothes. They will only serve to depress you in the future.

Put garments that need mending or cleaning into the basket. Set a time in the next week to get them done (or take them to a professional). Assess each piece and make sure they are worth the effort before you invest your time and money in them.

As for the "unfinished outfits," remember this:

If you can't pair it, you won't wear it.

Determine whether or not each article is worth keeping, shopping for, or spending money on to make it into an outfit. If it is, snip a little piece of fabric from an inside seam of the garment and put it on a safety pin. Keep the swatches in your wallet in a clear slot where you can see them. The next time you shop, it will help you recall what you need to focus on finding for your wardrobe.

Do not put the items back in the closet until they are wearable. Temporarily park them in another closet. In the end, don't be surprised if the majority of this category ends up at a rummage sale. Often, we have good intentions for these clothes, but seldom the time to fuss with them.

As for the articles you do not want to work with, put them in a bag to give away.

Keepers

These are the clothes that we love and wear often. They are the things that generate compliments and make us feel fabulous. As you sort through these components, spread them out on your bed and analyze each one. Ask yourself: Does it need replacing? Why is it a favorite? Is it the color, the style, the fabric, or the fit? Consider duplicating it in a different color, or make note of the fabric and replicate it in another piece. Note these things on paper to help you plan for future shopping endeavors.

We will return to this group when we are done sorting.

Losers

This is self explanatory: Losers are anything we wish we didn't own, including the following:

- Things that don't fit and can't be altered.

- Colors that make us look drained.

- Anything that is uncomfortable, physically or mentally.

- Something we wear once a year just so we can keep it there.

- Slacks that have been just a little too small for the last three years.

- Excess ratty weekend clothes. How many shirts do we need to paint in?

- Dead lingerie (bra straps that slip, exhausted elastic, old underwear).

- A notch down in quality from what we are currently wearing.

Another helpful question to ask is: Does it look as good on me as it did when I first bought it?

To sum it all up: **If it doesn't delight you, dump it**.

Put all of the "losers" into the bag along with the finders you didn't want and get them out of the house. These clothes can be handled in one of the following ways:

1. **Recycle**: Take the exceptional, in style, stain-free pieces to a consignment store and deposit the money into your clothing budget for next year.

2. **Rummage**: Price the clothes as you box them up and sell them to the neighbors. One woman's junk is another woman's fashion statement.

3. **Re-gift**: Donate them to mission groups, women's shelters; the Goodwill, and the Salvation Army can put them to good use.

If you are the type of person who is always saving her clothes for special occasions or resists wearing them for fear of ruining them—stop it! They are only clothes and are meant to be worn and enjoyed. Life is short.

Weepers

Weepers are our "sentimental journey" category. These are the things we can't bear to part with but never wear:

The dress worn for a sister's wedding

The designer suit we spent a bundle on

The hand-crocheted sweater Aunt Edith made

This category will include anything you have an emotional attachment to in relation to a time or event in your life. Things we don't wear have no right to be in our everyday closets. Put these treasures in a box and transport them out of the bedroom. Store them in a trunk up in the attic and visit them once a year.

Other "trophies" include our collection of t-shirts that have been acquired through sports and promotions like charities, marathons, and advertising ploys. Three to five "fun" t-shirts are plenty. Keep the ones you need, and give the rest away or cut them into rags. If you don't, they can mysteriously reappear in the closet.

Jeans have an emotional pull of their own. They make us feel young, skinny, or comfortable. Like old friends, they are hard to let go of. There are those we hold onto in the hope that one day we'll fit into them again. Ladies, if it's been longer than a year, get real. The fact is, if we do lose the weight, chances are they won't fit us the same as they once did. Unfortunately, our bodies change with time and gravity. When you lose the weight, reward yourself with a new pair.

It can be very difficult to let go of the "weepers," but to achieve the goal of an efficient wardrobe, sacrifices must be made.

■ MAINTAINING ORDER

By now, you should be facing an empty closet. If this is not the case, analyze what is left behind. Has it become a storage shed for stashing miscellaneous things? Clutter complicates life. Find a new home for these treasures and reclaim your space. Keep only wearable articles of clothing and accessories in the closet, nothing else.

Take a minute to dust and vacuum the vacant space before filling it again. Pull out the new hangers you bought and go to your "keeper" pile.

Start by organizing clothes by function. Hang all your shirts together, then all your slacks, then all your jackets, and so on. Take it a step further and color-code the categories going from the lightest (white, cream, beige) to darkest You won't have to "scan" the entire closet when looking for an item of a specific color.

Place sweaters/sweatshirts, three to a stack, on shelves where they remain visible to prevent a jumbled mess later. Scarves should also be on a shelf, layered in clear storage boxes.

Designing your closet in this manner will help you discover new ways to coordinate outfits.

Hang all the hangers on the rod backwards when switching seasonal clothes so that the open part of the hook is toward you. Once you've worn something, flip the hanger in the correct direction, so the open end is away from you. If you chose a garment and don't get beyond your bedroom door with it, replace it in the backward position again. At the end of the season you will know which clothes you wore and which ones you didn't, making it easier to sort next time.

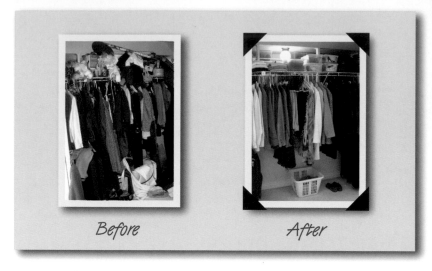

Before   *After*

With a few short hours and a plan in hand, your closet can move from a "before" to an "after"—setting you free from the stress of clutter and opening a world of new wardrobe options with what you already own!

Develop a "Grab and Go" Wardrobe

If time and energy are valuable commodities in your life, I suggest hanging complete outfits on one hanger. For example: the slacks with a t-shirt draped over them, the jacket around the hanger with earrings in the pocket, and a necklace and socks wrapped around the neck of the hanger. Create three to five hangers with various ensembles to suit your lifestyle needs. The next time you have to dress on the run, simply grab what you need and go.

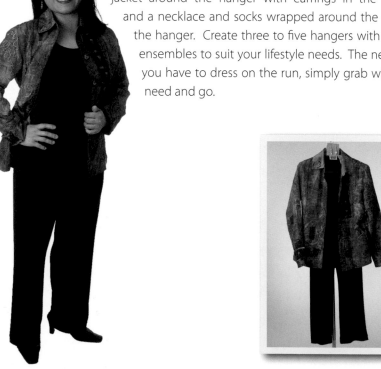

Off Season Storage

There are several viable options for clothing that needs to be stowed for a season or two:

1. **Utilize space under the bed** with large flat boxes. If the bed is too low, put a couple of bricks under the legs to elevate it.

2. **Use suitcases** to store off-season clothes since vacation is the most likely time you will need them again.

3. **The local drycleaner** will clean and store clothing for a nominal fee.

4. **Large plastic containers** or garbage cans with lids work well for storing things in the basement or garage and will help keep out moths and moisture.

Label each container as to the contents. As you put them away, make a note on the calendar at the start of next season as to what items are needed for the coming year. For example: the navy turtleneck that wore out, the leather gloves that were lost, or the black pants you outgrew. Shopping for the coming season will be much easier.

Future Investments

Keep a notebook and pen handy in your closet. The next time you are getting dressed and suddenly realize that you do not have the right undergarment, belt, or shell to make an outfit work, write it down. Before leaving on your next shopping trip, tear the page off and take it with you. This will prove to be a valuable reminder and help build a workable wardrobe.

Whenever you add something new to your closet, rotate out something old or rarely worn.

CLOSET CONFESSIONS

Closets are great places to hide things. We can store unnecessary items, stash unwanted pieces, or bury regrettable purchases. Closets become our secret hoarding places. Yet, the more useless things we hang onto, the less space we have for the essentials.

Our minds are emotional closets. How many worthless things are we storing there that are using up valuable space? As I open the doors of my own mind, I am amazed at how much junk I have collected over the years.

I find that I pull out and try on these unattractive things when my self-esteem dips.

I have a costly suit made of material from past situations that caused me "justifiable" anger. It's lined with 100% pride and stitched together with unforgiveness. I bought it because, at the time, it felt good. When I wear this suit, it looks sharp and dramatic. But underneath it is cold and uncomfortable. I should have paid attention to the label:

For if you forgive men when they sin against you, your Heavenly Father will also forgive you. But if you do not forgive men their sins, your Father will not forgive your sins. (Matthew 6:14-15)

A heavy coat has been hanging in my closet, on and off, for years. It's one I made myself, woven with yarns of disobedience, mistakes, and poor choices. I pull it out when the storms of fear begin to rage. The purpose is to protect myself and those I love from the harsh elements of life. When I try to dress my family in it, they despise my good intentions. The weight is so overwhelming it drags me down. This garment of guilt never seems to fit anyone. I gave it to Jesus years ago, but I keep taking it back again, despite the fact that his receipt clearly stated:

I will cleanse them from every sin they have against me and will forgive all their sins of rebellion against me. (Jeremiah 33:8)

There are a couple of gaudy accessory pieces that I've held on to for decades. Jewelry that is so flashy and ostentatious one has to look through squinted eyes to see it. Jealousy and envy would occasionally accessorize my thoughts when others were doing better or accomplishing more than I was. These gems seemed dazzling at first and were fun to wear. But like most cheap jewelry, with time the polish began to diminish. After close examination an imprint revealed it's true substance:

For where you have envy and selfish ambition, there you will find disorder and every kind of evil practice. (James 3:16)

No wonder this closet was such a mess. I acquired all of these things for the wrong reasons: selfish ambition and pride. At the time I thought they were stylish and made me look good. Instead, the wardrobe and accessories I chose were unbecoming, unflattering, and *ugly*.

Hasty mending of my own accord did nothing to enhance their condition. Surrendering them to Jesus was the only enduring solution. Because of Christ's sacrifice and promise of forgiveness I can discard these hideous belongings. He will dispose of them as if they never hung in my closet. He has a beautiful garment ready for me to wear sewn with threads of humility and love. Jesus paid the price.

I, even I, am he who blots out your transgressions, for my own sake, and remembers your sins no more. (Isaiah 43:25)

7 SIMPLE STEPS

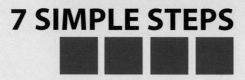

1. Survey your closet situation and determine your storage and hardware needs. List them.

2. Set aside a day on the calendar to organize your closet.

   Date: _____

3. Enlist a friend or get a video camera to help with wardrobe assessments.

4. Collect all of your organizing supplies before the big day.

5. Purchase a full-length mirror for your bedroom if you don't already own one.

6. Make a list of clothing items and accessories to complete fragmented outfits.

7. Decide to forgive someone and be forgiven today. Pray for God's help. When an unseemly incident knocks at the door of your memory, lock it out and remember how God has lovingly forgiven you.

Additional resources:
The New Messies Manual by Sandra Felton
Simplify Your Life by Marcia Ramsland
website: www.Flylady.net

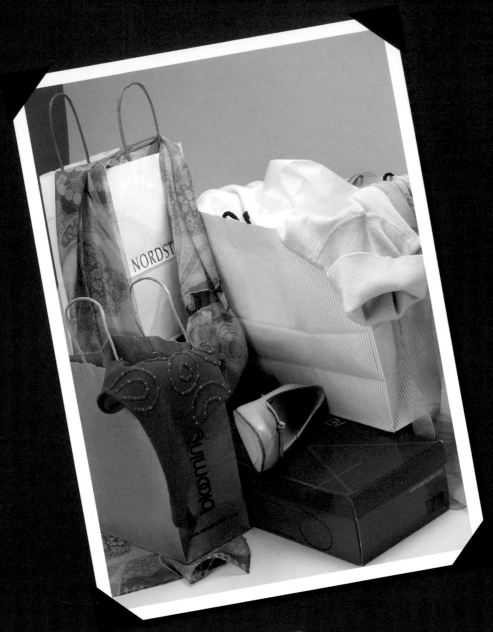

Simply Beautiful

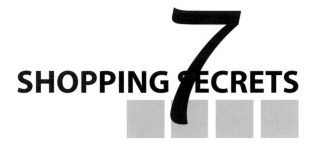

SHOPPING 7 SECRETS

So many stores, so little time... energy... and money.

When it comes to shopping, most women are in one of two camps; they *love* it, or they *hate* it. As a personal shopper who earns a living scouring the gamut of garments, I understand the many frustrations of trying to pull together a wardrobe. My clients often lament with dissatisfaction in the whole shopping experience, and with good reason. Their anti-retail rationale includes the following:

"I can never find my size."

"The stores don't carry styles that are flattering for my figure."

"I don't have the time."

"Clothes have gotten so expensive."

"What I have in my closet looks better than what's on the racks at Saks."

"I've put on a few pounds, and shopping depresses me."

"The colors and styles this season are ugly."

Can you relate? Help is here! Whether you shop for the sport of it, or consider the outing sheer torture, having a plan and knowing some basic rules will help you shop successfully. These ideas will equip you for wise wardrobe decisions and ease the stress of exploring uncharted territory.

■ THE GOLDEN RULES OF SHOPPING

Rule #1: LOVE IT OR LEAVE IT

Buy what you love, if you're not wild about it, don't be lured into buying clothing or accessories just because they've been marked down. The best way to test your purchase motive is to ask, "Would I pay full price for this?" The price will often appear more attractive than the piece. It takes discipline to restrain from buying for the sport of it.

Definition of a sale: A huge event held by a retailer to get everything out of their store and into your closet.

We all like to think of ourselves as savvy shoppers who know how to invest wisely in our wardrobes. First, we will scout out the "50 percent off" racks, then gleefully grab an armload of clothes and head to the dressing room. After trying on a few articles, the justification process begins to emerge; we frantically want something to work out. We reason: "Even though the color isn't very flattering, it does fit, and I might not find anything else." Or, "Well, it's a little tight, but I love the texture of the fabric and the tone of blue. I can hang it on my closet door and use it as my motivation to lose ten pounds."

Wake up! If the color doesn't flatter you now, it never will. To most women, if the color isn't right, it's all wrong – whether you are talking about furniture, cars, or clothing. And, future weight loss is *not* a safe criteria to use when buying tight-fitting clothes. You may drop the pounds, but it doesn't mean the garment will fit your new proportions.

Don't buy anything on sale that you would not have considered paying full price for in the first place.

Rule #2: SHOP FOR COLOR FIRST, STYLE SECOND

Suppose there was a treasure hunt contest at your local mall with a grand prize of a $1000 shopping spree. You choose the challenge:

a) Find twenty different blouses with a V-neckline
OR
b) Collect twenty different garments in the color green.

Unless you are color blind, most would pick the green. Our eyes work like radar detectors when honing in on a hue because it's faster to spot a color than a style.

Do you know what colors look best on you? Wearing the right colors can make you look absolutely radiant! Having your colors analyzed by a professional image consultant will yield long term rewards: clothes that mix and match easily, makeup that looks great with your natural coloring and a confidence that comes from wearing shades in harmony with your God-given beauty.

Each person has a set or "season" of colors that complement their eyes, hair and skin tone. People with yellow skin tone, reddish or golden hair color and eyes with brown, green or amber in them tend to look best in warm colors: peach, rust, caramel, gold, green, etc… If your skin has a bluer undertone (dark black, pale white, pink), and your hair is very dark, white or has ash tones, and your eyes are blue, black brown or blue-green, you may find the cool palate of colors work best: blue, pink, burgundy, violet, gray, etc…

This picture shows the dramatic difference that color can make especially when pulled together using makeup that complements your natural beauty.

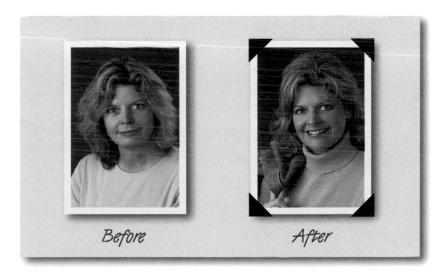

Before   *After*

Lisa glows when wearing bright colors that bring clarity to her skin tone.

Knowing your best colors and having an idea of what shade(s) you want to add to your wardrobe will save you hours of shopping, not to mention energy spent in the dressing room. With a trained eye you will be able to glance over racks and easily zero in on your target. The trick is to stay focused on what you are looking for.

Rule #3: DETERMINE COST PER WEARING

Money spent is money spent. We are most vulnerable when it looks like we are getting a good deal on something. Temptation can cause a mental lapse, like the old "buy one, get one free" sale. In a weak moment I have succumbed to purchasing two cheap sweaters only to have them fade and pill after the first washing. In retrospect I knew I should have put that $20 toward the beautiful cashmere sweater I adored and felt delicious in. But it's hard to justify spending all that money at the time.

While some price tags would give anyone sticker shock, for many of us it's difficult to sort out whether or not a piece of clothing is worth the investment. There is one tried and true way to look at a garment and assess it's value—cost per wearing. For example: a glitzy evening dress that can be used only for very formal occasions and may get worn a grand total of two times. At the sale price of $150, that comes out to be a pricey $75 per debut. Instead, consider using that $150 to purchase a good quality, navy blazer—one dressy enough to wear to work and casual enough to wear with jeans as an outside coat. It will get worn hundreds of times over the years.

Buy less and buy the best

Each time you don that classic jacket, cost divides, and you can wear it for as little as $1 a day.

Navy Blazer $100.00
—————————————   *= $1 or less a day*
   100+ times worn

Evening Dress $100.00
—————————————   *= $50 per wear*
      2 times worn

It pays to take the time to factor in a garment's wearability relative to your lifestyle. This technique is a valuable tool when trying to explain to your logically-minded spouse why you had to spend so much on one piece: it's an investment.

Rule # 4: IF IT DOESN'T FIT, IT ISN'T "IT"

I think the most frustrating aspect of shopping for most women is finding clothes that fit properly. Not only is it time-consuming, but it can be depressing as well. Our bodies are ever changing as parts shift, and in some cases, expand or contract. This is why it is imperative to always try on a garment before purchasing it.

There are a few shortcuts that can be taken in this process. First, before you venture out to shop, survey what is in your closet that fits you well now. Note the size *and* the brand. Different manufacturers have different standards for fit; when you find one that's in harmony with your body shape, stick with it.

Second, learn how to measure up a size before hauling something into the dressing room. When you shop, wear clothes that fit you correctly. They can be your biggest asset in making assessments without trying everything on. Once you are in the store and have found a contender, hold the garment up to your body. Match the shoulder seams to the edge of your shoulders; do they line up evenly on both sides? Run the sleeve line down your arm: Is the length right? It's a lot like playing with paper dolls, only you are the doll, and the clothes are fabric. When checking the size on a pair of slacks or jeans, zip and button them and hold them up in front of you. Match the side seams at the waist and hip area to the ones you are wearing, stretching them across your abdomen: Are they the same width across or an inch too small? If there is an inch difference, adjust by going up or down one size.

This technique also works well when shopping for others, such as a reluctant child or spouse. If you can't bring in the person, bring the garment that fits them best and use it as your pattern.

When you finally graduate to the dressing room, evaluate. Put the garment on and fasten all the buttons, zippers, snaps, and hooks. Stand squarely in front of the mirror, checking the front, sides, and back. There should be no indication of stress or wrinkling, no binding, gapping, and pulling at the buttonholes. Your slacks should not be "smiling" across the crotch. Move in it and ask yourself, "Does my body feel at ease?" If it does, it's for you; if not, move on.

Rule #5: NEVER BUY A STEP LOWER IN QUALITY

Debbie was a diehard "Liz Claiborne" customer. Not only did the designer clothing line fit her well, but she loved the vibrant colors and felt attractive whenever she wore them. One day while shopping with her teenage daughter, she ambled into a discount clothing store where everything was $10 or less. Debbie found a bright red, cotton t-shirt for $5. Who could resist? It was perfect for the barbecue they were invited to that night. She brought it home and paired it up with her white Liz slacks, silver earrings, and light leather slip-on shoes. A glance in the mirror before dashing out the door revealed that something was not right. The shoddy workmanship of the shirt cheapened the overall look of the outfit. At the end of the evening when she got home, Debbie noticed a red hue on the waistband of her pants. The dye from the $5 shirt had ruined her $50 slacks!

Sometimes "deals" can turn out to be duds, especially when the pieces we purchase are a downgrade from the overall quality we are accustomed to wearing. Stay at the same level as your prevailing look, or move up a notch. A step down can quickly become unattractive and unworn.

Downgrade some of your clothing at the end of the season. Older professional clothes become "better casuals," casuals can become "grungies" for painting in, etc.

■ To Buy or Not to Buy

I have to admit, there have been times in my life when I've shopped with the mentality of the bumper sticker "The Woman with the Most Clothes Wins!" Why? In some cases it was because I would bring home items that were "good enough," and later discover something better in another store. Or, there was the unique blouse I bought because it had a "different look," only to realize later that it was so different that I never felt comfortable wearing it.

Have you ever looked longingly at a dress in a store and left without buying it? The next week you find yourself reflecting on the beautiful style and how well it flattered your figure. You question whether or not you should have splurged and finally decide to go back and get it, only to find that the dress is gone. How disheartening! Some days I can let it go by saying "God didn't want me to have it now," but other times I simply regret not going with my instincts.

So how does one go about making that final decision? Is there any way to shop for clothes without experiencing buyer's regret? Yes! A technique I call **"Four Stars."** When used correctly, this method will eliminate costly mistakes and help you build a functional and flattering wardrobe. Begin by asking yourself the following questions concerning the item you are deliberating on:

⭐ **Does this piece complement me in three ways?**

1. The style reflects my *personality.*

2. The fit enhances my body *shape.*

3. The color flatters my *features.*

⭐ **Will this piece go with three different things I already own?**

Consider the garment's flexibility for mixing and matching with your current wardrobe.

⭐ **Can I wear this piece to three different events?**

Versatility is important when it comes to factoring in how often you will be able to use it.

⭐ **Can this piece be worn three years *stylishly?***

Often if a garment is on a sale rack, it may be going out of style in the near future.

If you answer "yes" to the first question, you're on your way to success. A "yes" answer to two out of the three remaining questions means you can feel confident about your purchase. If you got all four stars, go for it—it was made for you!

■ Strategic Planning

Now that you know the rules, let's move on to a plan of action. Are you serious about building a flattering wardrobe that will work for you financially? Do you want ensembles that make you look and feel fabulous? If so, a little discipline and strategy will go a long way in making for a successful hunting trip. The first step is to take inventory of what is currently hanging in your closet and tucked in your dresser drawers.

Have you ever planned to prepare a new recipe for a big dinner party and gotten to the grocery store without your list? It's frustrating as your mind turns to mush, and you can't seem to visualize what was printed on that recipe card, let alone the items that were lacking in your cupboards. Taking inventory and making a list are key ingredients to planning any successful shopping trip, whether to the grocery store or the mall. Know what you have and what you need. As the old saying goes, "We don't plan to fail, we fail to plan."

On that same note, I want to warn you about shopping for too many things at once. If building on what you have in your closet is your goal, choose one wardrobe centerpiece to work around, such as a favorite jacket or slacks that fit to a "T." Then focus on making one or two great outfits out of them. Shop only for what you will need in the next three months, not a year from now.

Bring along fabric snippets from clothes you own and want to build into ensembles. Put the swatches on a safety pin, and place them in a clear picture page in your wallet.

The second step is to set aside a full day to shop and save, or budget money, specifically for this endeavor. Consider doing the bulk of your seasonal wardrobe shopping in one twenty-four hour period. This is the most economical route to take. Why? Because if you desire a closet with clothing that you love to wear, you must focus on buying outfits instead of pieces. Little chinks of time spent here and there in the stores tempt us to purchase haphazardly. The results are a drained wardrobe account, as well as unmatched accessories and apparel items that stand alone, literally. If you want to do recreational shopping, save it for vacation or leave your money and credit cards at home.

▨ Accessory to the Crime

This is a shopping trip you will want to do alone or with an **honest** friend or relative who will shop for you. The focus has to be exclusively on **your** wardrobe, and not the needs of another person or project. You have a job to do with a tight deadline. Multi-tasking is not an option and will only complicate the process. Choose your accomplice wisely. I know of friends who become liabilities in the process of making wise wardrobe investments. They are the ones who don't have the heart to tell you how silly you look in an outfit *before* you buy it.

Timing Is Everything

When setting a date for your adventure, bear in mind your current needs. Are you looking for good deals? If so, try the last part of a season, the end of the month, or the day after a holiday. This is when retailers are trying to move merchandise out of the store quickly to do inventory.

Are you searching for the best selection for a certain time of year or event? Seasonal shopping means you have to have your act together about two months prior to the season you want to buy for. Shop in April for summer clothes, July for autumn, February for spring, and September/October for winter. If it is a wedding or formal affair, plan three to six months in advance and take advantage of after-event sales, January (New Year's), June (proms), and August (summer weddings).

Gearing Up

What you look like when you step foot into a mall can play a major role in what you ultimately end up purchasing. Haven't we all, at one time or another, attempted to shop in clothes that are comfortable and do nothing to complement our figure or face? While comfort is an asset when attempting a mission like this, it can also be a liability. Often if we don't take time to look our best before entering the glamorous world of fashion (the mall), we find that it is easy to purchase pieces that merely improve on what we started out with that morning.

For your convenience, here is a list of what to avoid:

What Not to Wear Shopping

1. Clothes with multiple buttons, ties, and zippers.

2. Layers of clothing, especially tight turtlenecks that are difficult to remove.

3. Slacks or jeans that are tight or have small ankle openings.

4. Shoes or boots that have to be laced or buckled up.

5. Excess accessories: scarves, dangly earrings, belts, or long necklaces.

6. Anything that makes you feel unattractive.

When shopping, wear clothes that are easy to get in and out of, to facilitate your trips to the fitting room.

Self-esteem can hit an all-time low when the sharply dressed salesperson ignores you to focus on her folding and straightening, neglecting your sighs and grunts. Then, after seeing all these beautiful people, you pass a tired, frumpy looking woman meandering in the next aisle and suddenly realize you're looking in a mirror. It does pay to dress up a bit. Put on your makeup, do your hair, and wear something that fits you and is flattering.

There have been occasions when I have pondered a purchase and thought, *what I'm wearing looks better than this outfit*, and back on the rack it goes! If I had dressed down that day, I would have probably bought it.

While looking good is important, one has to be comfortable. If not, you will find yourself tired and crabby before you make it to the halfway point of your day.

Stash your coat, gloves, and sunglasses in the car or a public locker when going into the mall. The less you have to carry around the better.

"Power shop" on your lunch hour when you are wearing an ensemble in need of accessorizing. It's easy and effective!

One other option to seriously consider when dressing to shop is to wear something that warrants help: a shirt that needs accessorizing, the vest that you love and doesn't go with anything you own, or ideally, the "centerpiece" you are going to work around to build your wardrobe. This will streamline the job and help you stay focused on making an outfit "come together."

Charting Your Course

Be prepared to start out early and eat a good breakfast. You'll need the energy. Plan to take some breaks in between stores, and schedule your lunch before or after the noon rush. In an effort to make this day the most efficient, the goal is to scout out the best deals first. Therefore, the strategy looks like this:

1. Consignment shops

2. Discount stores

3. Department stores

4. Specialty shops and boutiques

While not everyone is into consignment shopping, bear in mind that this is not your grandmother's thrift shop. Today's upper scale consignment stores carry high-end clothing lines with designer names and styles that are current with the trends. About 80 percent of my wardrobe is from consignment boutiques. The uniqueness of the clothes and the quality at discounted prices make me feel as though I can dress like a queen on a peasant's budget.

The next stop will be the discount stores. These include: TJ Maxx, Marshalls, Ross for Less, Loehmanns, DSW Shoes, Target, and similar stores. Here you will find a smorgasbord of brand name clothing and accessories at very reasonable prices. For example, if you are looking for a white cotton blouse, wouldn't you rather pay $19.99 at one of these places than $59.00 at a retail shop?

While at times this type of store can seem overwhelming, don't let the size and its warehouse appearance deter you. Start in the designer area. Use your eye to sort out color as you scan over the racks. Don't compromise on quality. There will be a mix of good and bad, first rate and cheap, and perfect and imperfect. Check the garment over carefully before making a final purchase.

On to the department stores—these cover a range from Nordstroms to Bloomingdales and Dilliards to Marshall Fields—depending on your own personal preference. Many of these retailers have special coupon sales or savings events that

If you need to replace a staple in your wardrobe (i.e. black slacks, navy blazer) never sacrifice comfort, quality or style for price. These are the tried and true requirements!

require some pre-planning. Do your homework before heading out, and check your local newspaper or call the store to find out what deals they are offering that day. If you hate to shop, consider using the personal shopper some of these stores provide at no cost.

When you enter a large store, start at the back of the clothing department by the sale racks and work your way forward to the mall or main entry. This will ensure that you haven't missed any bargains. Don't forget to take time to check out the accessory and shoe departments as well.

Last but not least, allow some time for the specialty shops and boutiques. This will include stores like Casual Corner, Chico's, and Ann Taylor, as well as the unique one-of-a-kind stores found in downtown areas. If you favor one of these types of shops and always seem to find something you love in them, start here first. The garment you buy here may end up being the new centerpiece you wish to build on.

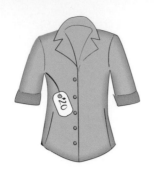

In the end, do not remove any tags or lose track of receipts until you have gone home and tried everything on again the next day. Introduce your new pieces to your existing wardrobe and make certain they are all going to get along well. Smile and take a deep breath. You now have a closet full of clothes, and things you *want* to wear.

■ Shopping Wisely

The ultimate shopping trip recorded in the Bible had to be the one where God gave King Solomon a blank check and said, "You can have anything you want, just ask and it's yours." What an awesome opportunity! Now if it were me, I might have requested happiness, health, love, riches, a long life, peace…my list could go on and on. But Solomon's simple request was for wisdom. (I Kings 3:5-14).

King Solomon asked for wisdom with a purpose in mind: To use it to guide God's people. He wasn't just shopping for himself when he made his plea. The Lord gave it to him in abundance and threw in riches and honor as an added bonus. The good news? This same wisdom that Solomon received is also available to us!

In James 1:5 it says:

If any of you lacks wisdom, he should ask God, who gives generously to all without finding fault, and it will be given to him.

We need to pray and ask for it. I would venture to say that this is a safe request. In the past, I have prayed for patience and ended up with stress-inducing moments that tested it. Then there was the time I prayed for self-control to stop raising my voice around my family and wound up with laryngitis for two weeks. I guess I should have asked for wisdom on what to pray for!

For the Lord gives wisdom, and from his mouth come knowledge and understanding. (Proverbs 2:6)

He *gives* us the wisdom, but *from his mouth* come knowledge and understanding. God's mouth is His Word, the Bible. We need to read it and search for understanding as if we are looking for hidden treasure (see Proverbs 2:4-5). How often do you go shopping for a specific clothing item, walk into the first store, and find exactly what you had in mind? Most seasoned shoppers know that this is highly unlikely. We need to be willing to put forth effort to find what we desire.

Have you ever known anyone who was intelligent and yet lacked common sense? A mind is a terrible thing to waste. By pursuing wisdom on our own and ignoring the Bible, we blindly stumble through life and lose out on the blessings that are hidden in its pages. When we earnestly seek knowledge through God's Word, we gain insight and discernment as to how to use that knowledge. Reading the Bible gives us an education that will last beyond a lifetime.

7 SIMPLE STEPS

1. Write out one golden rule that you will vow to use from now on when you shop. _____
   _____
   _____

2. Take inventory of your closet, and assess your current wardrobe needs.

3. Clip fabric from inseams of clothing that you intend to build on and put the swatches on a safety pin. Place the pin in the clear compartment at the front of your wallet.

4. List out the "Four Stars" questions on a 3 x 5 card, and carry it in your purse.

5. Pick a "centerpiece" to work around from your existing wardrobe.

6. Pull together the perfect shopping outfit from your closet, and set a date to shop strategically. _____
   _____
   _____

7. Seek the source of wisdom: God. Ask Him to give you knowledge and understanding. Open your mind and heart to His Word, and you will receive it abundantly.

Additional resources:
Dressing Like a Million Bucks by JoAnn Janssen and Gwen Ellis

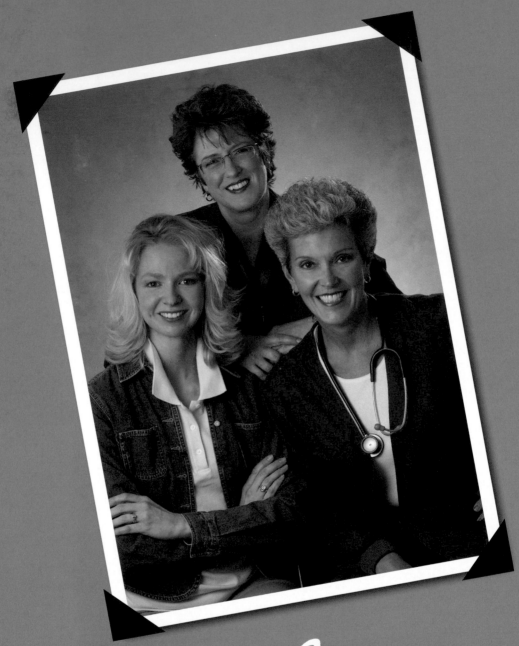

Simply Beautiful

PHASES **OF FASHION**

If nothing changes, then nothing changes.

Printed on a pink sheet of paper and posted on the locker room wall of the local health club, this quote stopped me cold in my tracks. Confused by its simplicity, I read it again. *If nothing changes, then nothing changes.* The intent was to encourage those of us who had hit a plateau in our weight and fitness endeavors to pursue new avenues of exercise. While I *do* like change occasionally, I am a creature of habit. I'm comfortable doing my routine of thirty-five minutes on the elliptical machine and lifting a few sets of hand weights. Sweating it out on a Nordic track or stumbling around in an aerobics class did not entice me, but alas, I too had to face reality; my scale had not moved for months.

It reminds me of life. Just when we get comfortable, something forces us to change, like it or not. From youth to maturity, childhood to motherhood, and jobs to careers, change is inevitable. If we don't adjust, like my scale, we too remain unmoved. As women, we will all play different roles throughout our lives. This chapter is written to help jump-start your wardrobe for whatever stage of life you are experiencing.

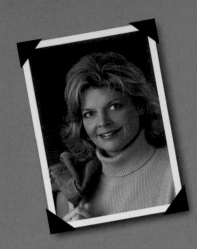

MULTI-TASKING MOM

All mothers are working mothers.

When you announced that you were going to have a baby, how many people said, "Your life is really going to change!" I don't know about you, but after a while, that little statement began to strike terror in my heart. What did they mean? Often it was followed with a little quip like, "your life will never be your own again." It sounded more like a warning than a word of encouragement!

While it's true to say that my life's schedule and priorities did change, I think the biggest surprise for me was how it affected my wardrobe and dressing style. I don't mean just maternity clothes (we adopted), but the whole "mommy thing" turned my classic business and high maintenance trousseau into "museum art" that merely hung in my closet. I'd open the door, gaze at it, and wearily reach down and pull my worn sweatsuit out of the clothes basket.

A few months into this new "career," I happened by a mirror. Who was that dowdy woman who looked like she hadn't seen sleep in years? I looked awful! The fact was that disguising the ravages of being overtired and under-dressed didn't hold much appeal; I felt exhausted! I had few "shopportunities" and when the prospect did arise, shopping for clothes with an infant was a rigorous workout. No longer was it the delightful "retail therapy session" it had once been.

"Beauty is all very well at first sight but whoever looks at it when it's been in the house three days?"
—George Bernard Shaw

With time I slowly got my act together, but I wish I had known before motherhood what I know now. I think I would have planned a little better. What follows are some of the best hair, makeup, and clothing tips for making motherhood a little more manageable.

The Pregnancy

This represents one of the few times in your life when you may have acquaintances and even total strangers tell you that you are "glowing." What a wonderful thing to hear, but somehow it doesn't make up for the multiple beauty problems the pregnant woman faces. Finding maternity clothes that do not make you look like a little girl, and shoes that are actually comfortable, can be a challenge. In a survey I conducted concerning the issue of favorite maternity wear, denim was the overall winner. One mom shared, "My favorite thing to wear when pregnant was, without a doubt, denim. I felt normal and in style with either jeans or a denim shirt or jean jacket over a cute t-shirt." Another said, "The best thing I had was a long denim skirt that could be casual or dressed up depending on the shoes. Investing in a good pair of jeans was also a smart idea."

To alter T-shirts and knit dresses without sewing: place front part of shirt over the end of your ironing board. Then using a hot, steam iron drag it slowly across the garment horizontally to stretch the fabric that covers the tummy area to make it bigger. After pregnancy, wash and dry on hot settings and shrink it back.

Here is a list of some transitional clothes that will help the woman with child continue to be the woman with style:

Maternity Style

1. A comfortable *denim* jumper or maternity dress

2. Cotton knit pants with long knit shirts

3. Bib overalls

4. Fabrics that are soft, non-shiny, and light-medium weight

5. Subtle, *unevenly* spaced prints

6. Maternity style dress in a fluid fabric

7. Men's shirts, sweaters, pajama pants, and boxers

8. One good pair of "in style" maternity jeans

9. Shoes that fit and feel great

10. A silky tunic and matching silky slacks

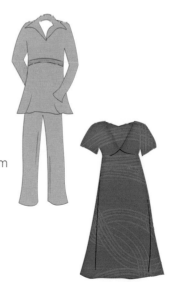

Queen-size pantyhose or knee highs are a good alternative to costly maternity hose.

Weight and body shape change considerably during the course of the pregnancy and the following year as well. For many expectant moms it is difficult to justify spending money on a wardrobe that will only fit for two or three months. Finding clothing styles that will cross over into your post pregnancy days and adapt to your changing body can be a challenge. Listed here are some key pieces that will adapt to weight fluctuation easily:

- A-line cut coats and dresses

- Chemise dresses (drop waist with blouse on top)

- No-waist dresses in soft, fluid fabrics

- Jumper dresses

- Long unconstructed jackets

- Swing jackets in drapable fabrics

- Raglan or full cut sleeves

- Knits

- Drawstring and elastic waistbands

Comfort is the top priority when it comes to dressing, but making yourself look and feel beautiful in ways that don't focus on your body weight is important as well. A leisurely scented bubble bath, pedicures, manicures, and getting a good haircut/color are all things you can control—unlike your growing tummy.

Consider swapping clothes among your pregnant friends; it will add some variety at no extra cost.

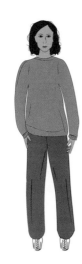

Motherhood with Style

When my kids were young, there was a line of clothing called "Garanimals." There were adorable mix-and-match pieces that facilitated formula dressing for the toddler. I've often thought this would be a good option for Moms as well. With children in the picture, clothes are no longer on the priority list. Guilt often enters in when budgets are adjusted to accommodate a new stay-at-home mom and an extra mouth to feed. Another issue is the time pressure factor. Who knew that once the kids were out of diapers we would still be trying to fit twenty-five hours into a day? Add to that the exhaustion factor of having to be "tuned in and turned on," 24/7, and "dressing with style" goes out the window!

Most at-home moms would reason that since they have no appearances to keep up, what's the sense? It's true that we all have days when fashion must take a back seat to housework, childcare, and chores. However, it's important to realize that even at home, *you become what you have on.* A regular routine of dressing in sloppy, oversized clothes not only affects your self-esteem, but also the approach you take to your work and your children's response to you. You need to "dress for success" at home by wearing cheerful, refreshing clothes.

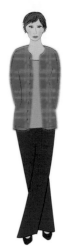

Try this experiment: Dress up a little more than normal around the house for a couple of days. Wear bright colors and clothes that fit you nicely but allow room for movement. Slap on some makeup and do your hair in a new way. Observe how your children and husband react. I think you'll be pleased with the results. Many women are surprised to find how just a few small outward changes can affect not only the attitudes of family members but their own as well.

I'm not expecting you to look radiant on a daily basis, but just tweaking your look ever-so-slightly can do wonders. A simple two-minute makeup job that includes mascara, blush, under-eye concealer and a dab of colored lipgloss can work wonders. Another trick is to try a new hairstyle. Update your cut, get a perm, do some highlights, or try bangs or "sideburns" for a change. If you are brave, experiment with some at-home hair care products. They're inexpensive, and you may learn a new skill in the process. Just be sure to follow all directions closely. It also helps to have an understanding professional hairdresser on standby. A new style can add zip to your "do-da" on days when you're feeling drab. That fresh, youthful feeling that comes from modifying your look is a real mood-lifter!

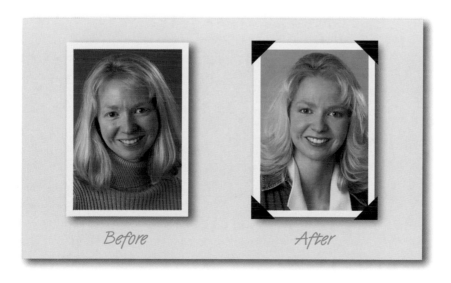

Before   *After*

Busy moms can look beautiful with just a touch of makeup, a natural hairstyle and a bright colored t-shirt.

Mothers need a wardrobe that combines style, comfort, and low maintenance. One way to achieve this is to keep the following basics in your closet:

The Casual Wardrobe

- Two pair of nice fitting (not tight) jeans

- Three collared shirts in bright colors

- A comfy skirt and knit sweater combination

- A longer, a-line soft denim or broom skirt

- A fashionable warm-up suit

- One to two pairs of corduroy or knit slacks with mix-and-match tops

- Two outfits for nights out or girlfriend get-togethers

- One pair of good leather loafers with matching socks

- One blazer that fits well and can be worn with jeans, slacks, or a skirt

I realize that a minimal wardrobe is going to differ for everyone, but this should give you a starting point. Jewelry and accessories are a bother, so for most moms I suggest having one pair of earrings you love and can sleep in, as well as a simple chain necklace with a pendant or cross that reflects your personality. Scarves are best left on the coat or dress you intend to wear them with. Secure them with a safety pin so they stay in place.

Real Contentment

"Happy is the man whose wife is content in the home." When my friend and mentor, Diane, uttered those words twenty-three years ago, little did I realize the impact they'd have on me over the decades to follow. At the time I was young and newly married. Life was good. I had the attention and admiration of my husband, a house filled with new gadgets and gifts from our wedding, and a title I'd sought after relentlessly for years, "Mrs." Home was a happy and satisfying place.

But the human desire for approval, possessions, and position is seldom quenched for long. As time progressed, life changed. Craig began working double shifts to meet the demands of his construction business and keep the bills paid. New things became old, and being a married woman often meant sitting home alone at night. If idle hands are the devil's workshop, then idle minds must be his control center. I wasted my evenings watching primetime soap operas and perusing fashion magazines—both fertile breeding grounds for materialistic wants and unrealistic romantic desires. Talking to others led me to believe that everyone else had a far better life.

Ah, then came *my* ultimate solution: Children. Having kids would make our house a home and give us a stronger marriage. When the children came, so did the reality. I saw less of my husband and expected much more of him. Things went from bad to worse, and ultimately we ended up seeing a marriage counselor. The doctor pointed out that our focus needed to be on what we had rather than what we lacked.

This age-old problem of discontentment dates back to creation and the first sin recorded in the Bible. Eve had it all: a beautiful place to call home, a loving husband who only had eyes for her, and all the food she could eat without concern for fat grams or calories. Things were fine and dandy until that snake came along and pointed out what she *didn't* have—the freedom to eat of one particular tree in the garden. He beguiled her with a lie to add flavor to the fruit, and said that wisdom would be hers if she would eat of it. She succumbed, and her contentment was irreversibly shattered.

The snake in our lives is the same Satan that tempted Eve, however, his tactics are more in tune with the 21st Century. He can subtly weave discontentment into our minds through the media, reading material, life's frustrations, or even a seemingly benign conversation. He twists our perspective by whispering lies in our ears, causing us to shift our attention from what we have to what we don't have. Whether it is where we live, who we live with, or what we do, our level of satisfaction affects not only us, but those we love and encounter each day.

Contentment is not a gift, but a choice. If you are struggling with wants and dissatisfaction in your life, ask God to remove those desires and teach you contentment. Only He can do this; He is all you need.

I lift up my eyes to the hills—where does my help come from? My help comes from the Lord, the Maker of heaven and earth. (Psalm 121:1-2)

This is an ongoing process and I must constantly remind myself to be "the wife content in the home." Repeating I Timothy 6:6 has helped keep my focus clear:

"But godliness with contentment is great gain."

7 SIMPLE STEPS

1. Invest in two pieces of comfortable, denim clothing.

2. Get one pair of shoes that fit and feel great on your feet.

3. Unwind with a pedicure, manicure, or bubble bath once a week.

4. Treat yourself to a new hairdo that is conducive to your lifestyle as a mom.

5. Throw out all ratty, unattractive "home clothes" that make you feel dumpy.

6. Use color and a touch of makeup to bring life to your daily look.

7. Remember, contentment is a choice. Be happy and stay focused on the "haves" and forget the "have nots."

Additional resources:
Facts of Life and Other Things My Father Taught Me by Lisa Whelchel
The Busy Mom's Guide to Prayer by Lisa Whelchel
websites: www.Hearts-at-home.org
              www.Momsintouch.org
              www.Mops.org

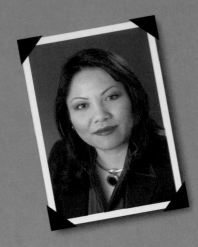

THE POLISHED PROFESSIONAL

"While clothes do not make the woman they certainly have a strong effect on her self-confidence —which I believe does make the woman."

—*Mary Kay Ash*

Whether doing a church presentation, attending a parent-teacher meeting, or applying for a job, how we look will influence those around us. Looking our best not only builds self-confidence both personally and professionally, but also projects a level of professionalism to those with whom we interact. Learning to dress for respect and using discretion in the process is essential to a winning wardrobe. Each of us, regardless of age, life stage, or occupation, will have occasions where projecting authority and competence are important.

Volumes of books have been written on this subject over the years, but none had more impact than John T. Molloy's bestseller in the mid-1970's entitled, *"Dress for Success."* In his book, Molloy touts the importance of first impressions and presents research on how people were perceived by strangers based on the style of clothing they chose. One study cited ten different decisions that could be made about us based on our appearance. This list includes things like our economic level, education, heritage, trustworthiness, level of sophistication, and moral character. It is interesting to note that one rarely alters that initial impression.

The Interview

Nowhere are first impressions more critical than at a job interview. While working as a staffing consultant for an employment agency, this became quite evident. My training and work as "the interviewer" gave me insight into the power of appearance and how it is assessed and interpreted in the business world. Only 20 percent of the people who came in seeking a job presented themselves appropriately for the initial meeting. Valuable time was spent coaching each on how to act and dress for a second level interview with perspective employers.

Competition in the job market is tough, and a polished professional image is your personal calling card. While judging a book by its cover is not something we should do spiritually, when *you* are "the book," you need a cover that will entice someone to consider looking at your content. Dressing for the part you intend to play will give you a distinctive edge. To look professional you must appear polished, put-together, and appropriate.

A polished look is one that is neat from head to toe. Carefully consider each of the following areas:

- **Hair**—be sure it is in style and professional. Long hair should be pulled back in a low ponytail or a French twist. Avoid ribbons, barrettes, and bows.

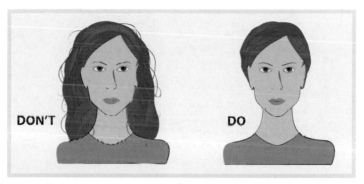

- **Make-up**—wear it, even if you normally don't. A little lipstick, blush, and mascara will give a fresh look and add sophistication. Keep the colors subdued, and avoid bright or frosted lipsticks and iridescent eyeshadows.

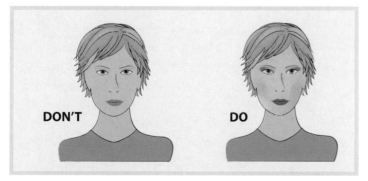

- **Accessories**—keep them at a minimum. The less of these you have on, the more credible you will appear. Though earrings give a finished look, they should be a medium size and not dangle. Necklaces, scarves, and leather goods should reflect quality.

- **Clothing**—must be neat, clean, and well-fitted. A suit or jacket are good choices for projecting authority and professionalism.

- **Hosiery**—make them sheer and matched to your skin tone. No snags, holes or runs, and no bare legs!

- **Shoes**—should be a neutral color, simple style in excellent condition. Colors like tan, taupe, black or brown are best. Avoid open toes, sandals, and boots. If the shoes are new, rough up the soles with sandpaper to prevent slipping.

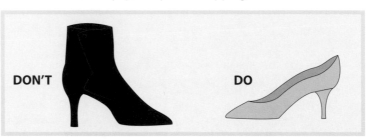

DON'T   DO

Unkempt or ill-fitting clothes will lower your perceived intelligence and make you look like you don't pay attention to details.

Give your interview outfit a trial run the night before a big day. Wear it for an hour, stand in it, walk in it, and sit in front of a mirror in it. Make certain there is no undergarment visibility and that buttons and hems are securely in place. Nothing should be too tight, too loose, or too low cut. One other consideration is to avoid wearing perfume or cologne. The scent can be distracting, and many people suffer from fragrance allergies.

DO

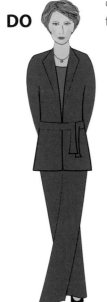

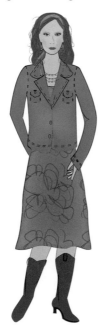

The personality of the company and the nature of work you are pursuing will play a key role in what you chose to wear. Ensuring that your wardrobe isn't outdated or inappropriate may require some research. Visit the potential work place before your interview to scope out what the management and the employees are wearing. Sitting discreetly in the parking lot in the morning to observe the standard of dress is another viable alternative. Dressing too conservatively for a creative job can be as detrimental as dressing wildly for the business sector. Do your homework!

Appearing "put-together" means that all elements of your look are in sync. When you appear intelligent and sophisticated, people tend to listen more carefully to your words.

DON'T

Making a Statement

There are times in our lives when we may need to look more or less powerful than we actually are. By gaining a better understanding of the hidden language of "lines and design," the correct use of curved or straight lines in clothing, details, and accessories can convey a message that speaks louder than words. Using straight lines and rigid fabrics helps us appear strong and forceful; conversely, curvy details and soft fabrics are inviting and non-threatening. These ideas can be easily implemented in all walks of life, whether business or personal.

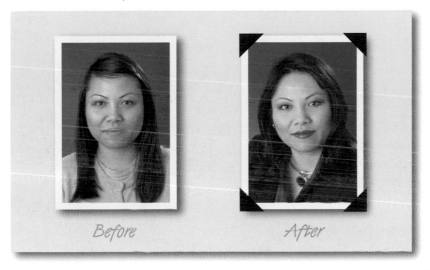

Before   After

To change Sinath's look from soft and shy to strong and sophisticated, we cut two inches off her hair, added bold makeup colors and replaced her soft lined clothing with a crisp tailored suit and shirt. Her new look is classy and refined yet still accentuates the youthful beauty of her face.

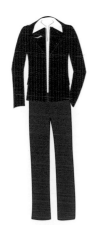

Begin by reviewing your agenda and those with whom you'll be involved. Are you asking for a raise? For donations? Having a parent-teacher conference? Next, consider how you want to be perceived. Do you prefer to be approachable and easy to talk to or maintain a more business-like attitude? For a more authoritative look, try the straighter and more structured lines of a tailored blazer. To appear more approachable and friendly, use curved, soft lines, like those in an angora sweater or soft cardigan.

Here is a breakdown of the two different styles.

AUTHORITATIVE	APPROACHABLE
Straight/vertical lines	Curved lines
Sharp edges	Soft edges
Crisp fabrics	Fluid fabrics
Fitted and tailored	Loose and flowing
Flat/smooth textures	Nubby/soft textures
Straight/geometric patterns	Rounded/swirl patterns
Solids	Prints
Notched/pointed collars	Rounded/shawl collars
Black, navy, charcoal, plum	Beige, light, or bright colors
Light and dark color combinations	Monochromatic, soft colors

For those occasions when you do not want to come across too extreme in either area, blending the two categories will help give a more balanced look when needed. For example, choose a straight-line, structured suit in a soft color and accessorize it with pearls. This subtle statement combines gentleness with an air of authority.

Business Casual

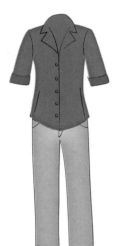

Most workplaces today have a dress code that is "business casual." Defining and executing it can be a challenge. Keep in mind that business casual means one step down from traditional attire, not "paint-the-house" or "wash-the-car" clothes. Outfits should be clean and pressed. Approach this look with the same care and thought you do when sending out correspondence. Dressing sloppy for work is no different than sending out a crumpled up business letter; neither is considered professional.

A textured jacket with a shawl collar or a quality polo shirt in a color that does not look "over-washed" with a pair of khaki slacks define business casual and are comfortable as well as professional. Another option is a neat denim shirt with corduroy pants. Jeans should be in top shape and not faded. Ask your employer if denim is acceptable before wearing it. Places of business often keep a published and updated listing of what is satisfactory and what is not.

It is important to carefully choose shoes and accessories that are well made, tidy and sharp, yet comfortable. Often people miss the mark and appear sloppy due to run-down accessory choices. You *can* appear neat from head to toe and still be comfortable.

Dressing Your Profession

Over the past decade, the pendulum of appropriate work attire has swung from one side to the other. The conservative suit was replaced by casual jeans and T-shirt, and is now heading back the other way. How can we begin to assess the "right way" to dress? Consider the job or profession that you are currently in or seeking. Most occupations can be categorized into one of three wardrobe styles:

- Conservative—management, financial services, secretarial, insurance, and marketing.

- Creative—advertising, entertainment, photography, fashion, and beauty.

- Caring—teaching, healthcare, counseling, childcare, and social work.

Conservative Professions

A traditional business wardrobe will best suit the conservative professional. Recognizing the impact of looking authoritative by choosing higher quality clothing and accessories, as well as using predominately "straight" lines will give a strong, credible first impression.

Working in management, finance, and legal professions necessitates a look that spells success. However, you don't have to be a millionaire to dress smart. Start shopping at quality consignment stores, outlet malls, and the designer sections of discount department stores such as TJ Maxx, Burlington Coat Factory, and Ross for Less. Strive for a mix-and-match wardrobe to give you a variety of looks with few pieces.

By dressing up, you make the client feel important. Use caution not to overdo it either way.

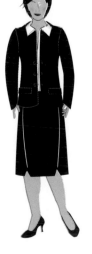

Basic Business Wardrobe

- **Two Suits:** One light to medium weight fabric in a dark color and one medium to heavy weight in a softer/neutral color. Choose simple uncluttered designs.

- **Two Blazers:** One solid basic color and one bolder color or a blend (e.g. tweed, herring bone, houndstooth).

- **Four Skirts/slacks:** Coordinate these with the jackets.

- **Five Blouses/shells:** White or beige; print; "signature colors" (see Chapter 1).

- **Sweater:** Cardigan, dark or neutral color.

- **Hose:** Beige, taupe, or off-black.

- **Two Pairs of shoes:** Basic pumps, neutral colors, varied heel heights, and in good condition (no scuffs, or heels that clack).

- **Jewelry and accessories:** Matched sets and quality material. Keep to a minimum.

- **Overcoat:** Simple, classic style that meets or exceeds hemline.

Begin by using two neutral colors as the core of your wardrobe, such as taupe and navy or dark olive and beige. Later you can easily add more colors and extra pieces to create interest with a vest, dress, or unique belt.

If you are in sales, a little fashion forwardness lets the client know that you are in tune with current trends. Always start by dressing your best—you need to sell yourself first. If your image and presentation are mediocre, the response from those you encounter will often be turned off and non-committal. However, don't overdo it, going to an industrial site to sell nuts and bolts in an Italian suit won't help you win friends and influence people. The client needs to be able to identify with you so they can trust you.

Creative Professions

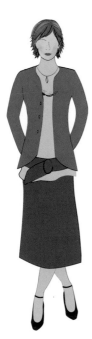

Women in creative professions ranging from retail to entertainment have a unique wardrobe challenge: combining credibility with creativity. While it is important to look polished and professional, it is equally important to demonstrate that you are open to new ideas and not afraid to experiment. This means artfully adding originality and imaginative flair to the "Basic Business Wardrobe."

Signature pieces make a strong statement. Bold necklaces, unusual scarves, or a distinctive style can express your personality and set you apart from others. This is exceptionally effective when you are in a competitive business or call on the same clients repeatedly. While working as a receptionist for a corporation, I remember one particular salesman, Bob, who had his own signature style. Bob wore bow ties, but he didn't stop there. He wore socks that matched his ties. I don't recall how successful Bob was, but I never forgot him. The moral of the story is: be certain your memorable impression is a favorable one.

If you look sharp, people will think you are sharp. Stay with the trends and avoid fads. Trends come in slowly and influence everything from fashion to architecture and interior design. They slowly evolve from what people are currently interested in—a movie, an event, culture, or economics—just to name a few. Modified shoulder pads, retro looks, and animal prints have proven to be long-term trends. Plastic baubles, neon colors, and matted faux fur are fads. Fads tend to come in quickly on the scene and are usually extreme. In other words, they are in one year and out the next. For further information on trends, check out www.projectsolvers.com. This is a wonderful resource for websites and publications that are design related.

If your hair and glasses look outdated, people will assume that your ideas are outdated as well.

Focus your attention on maintaining an image that reflects your talent, current trends, and creativity. Take into account the clients or employer you are working for and use the lines and designs that will make them feel comfortable and confident about you. Finally, make sure your ensemble is "put-together" and stylish.

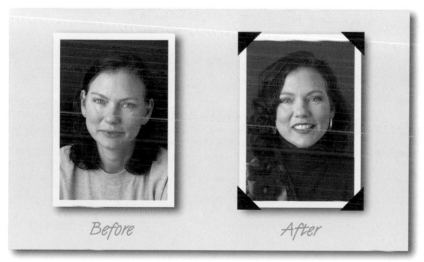

Before   After

Crystal's beautiful, warm coloring is accented by the rich brown sweater and bright scarf that lends a creative edge to her outfit.

Caring Professions

Caring people are busy people. Many give of themselves above and beyond the call of duty. These serving professions can often be draining— emotionally, mentally, and physically. They run the gamut of occupations from social and healthcare workers to teachers, missionaries, and counselors.

Choose seasonless clothes—pieces you can wear year-round: light weight wools, sturdy cottons, and silks.

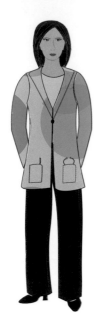

The demanding nature of people-oriented jobs requires a wardrobe that is functional, versatile, and comfortable.

From a functional point of view, simplicity is essential. Keep unnecessary details and accessories to a minimum. Consider the type of activity your job requires. If you are working with children or caring for the sick, a dangly necklace or scarf can be a nuisance when you lean over to give assistance. This doesn't mean eliminating accessories, but rather, choosing pieces that stay put. Try unique pins, chokers, or necklaces that are 14–18 inches long, and secure scarves with safety pins. If you are toting around tools of the trade, choose pockets from which you can easily get your hands in and out.

Working with a wide range of ages, or playing different roles within the same job, means a versatile wardrobe will be a good investment. Teachers may need to come across as authoritative with students but more approachable when dealing with parents, and in some cases vice-versa. The same can be said for people in childcare and counseling. Keep a soft, structured blazer in a dark color such as black or navy on hand for a quick change. Add a pair of slacks and a light color blouse with a collar to coordinate with the jacket, and you will project power and poise.

Fostering trust is as important as maintaining authority. You need to look caring and attentive, not intimidating. Putting people at ease is the first step in getting them to open up to you. Let your personality shine through in soft or bright colors, prints, and unusual accessories which will help initiate conversation. Soft fabrics and light shades communicate understanding and have a calming effect. Use the "Approachable" and "Authoritative" lists to further guide you in adjusting your wardrobe.

Shop for comfortable clothes and shoes late in the day.

Comfort is of the utmost importance. Clothing that binds, pulls, or shifts the wrong way when you move is not only an aggravation, but also a distraction. The challenge is finding pieces that feel *and* look good. Comfort is often equated with oversized, dowdy, or sloppy clothes. Can clothing be comfortable and flattering? Yes! Here are some basic guidelines to help you look and feel your best:

- Buy clothes that fit. Oversized pants and shirts look frumpy and unprofessional. Clothes that are too tight when trying to move or sit down will make you miserable. Scale clothing to your size and height.

- Invest in comfortable shoes. Quality material that cradles your feet should be top priority. Happy feet are vital to the rest of your body feeling agile and energetic.

- Choose fabrics that can be laundered, don't pill up and feel good next to your skin; like cottons, knits and fleece. Pre-washed garments will be your safest bet.

- Keep quality in construction a priority. Spending more on a well-made garment that has finished seams and good construction pays off in the number of times it gets worn.

- Pair a fitted top piece with a roomy bottom piece, or just the opposite. The fitted piece should be body conscious but not tight. The loose piece needs to stay put but allow you to move with ease.

Remember, comfort rules, but not at the expense of neatness and professionalism. The overall idea of professional dressing is to convey credibility and instill confidence. Or, as my father used to tell me when I was young, "Try to look and act like you knowed somethin'." Dad wasn't terribly eloquent, but he did get his point across!

Stressing for Success

Mother Theresa was once asked, "How can you bear the load without being crushed by it?" Her response was simple and to the point, "I am not called to be successful, but faithful."

The load a working woman carries day in and day out is a heavy one and to some, more of a burden. Trying to maintain balance in all facets of life is a constant juggling act. Combine this with client and employer expectations, scheduling demands, and a desire to do your best, and you have a formula for stress. How does one carry the burden without being crushed?

The answer can be found in the Bible:

Whatever you do, work at it with all your heart, as working for the Lord, not for men, since you know that you will receive an inheritance from the Lord as a reward. It is the Lord Christ you are serving. (Colossians 3:23, 24)

We all have different motives for doing a job well from start to finish. In the secular world, the motive might be climbing the ladder of success with a goal to be powerful, independently wealthy or even "the best." In such a case, motive begins with "M" and ends with "E," making the focus "ME." In a life totally given over to Christ, our motive shifts from one's self to Him. For whom are we working? The end of the Colossians verse makes it clear: *"It is the Lord Christ you are serving."* He's the only one we should seek to please.

Keeping perspective means that making decisions concerning priorities and time management need to be viewed in light of God's purpose for our lives. The only way to maintain a stress-free work environment is to make an appointment to meet with "the Boss" on a daily basis and ask for His direction. Throughout the day I call on Him for guidance while interacting with clients and their unspoken needs; for help in setting my speaking agenda for the coming months; and even what to fix for supper. I count on His direction to serve as a safety net as I follow Him and walk the balance beam of life.

So when your employer tells you you're staying for mandatory overtime, your computer shuts down for the third time in one day, or your cranky co-worker belittles you in front of your supervisor; consider it an opportunity for growth. Don't be a doormat, but be willing to let God use you and your faithfulness to influence others.

Faithfully working for the Lord, whether in ministry or in the secular world, reaps a reward that far outweighs what we can attain on this earth. The benefits include a paycheck of inner peace and joy, the best insurance policy you can get, and a retirement plan that is out of this world!

Therefore we also have as our ambition, whether at home or absent, to be pleasing to him. (II Corinthians 5:9 NAS)

7 SIMPLE STEPS

1. Review your overall image and ask, "Is it polished, put-together, and professional?"

2. Choose suits that cross over seasons or can be worn year-around.

3. Update your hair and glasses as needed.

4. Put together one "power" outfit using authoritative lines.

5. Use curved lines and soft fabrics to create one "approachable" ensemble.

6. Follow the accessory rule: "The less you have on the more credible you'll appear."

7. Keep your mind focused on Who you really work for.

Additional resources:
The Purpose Driven Life by Rick Warren
Godly Business Woman Magazine
www.godlybusinesswoman.com

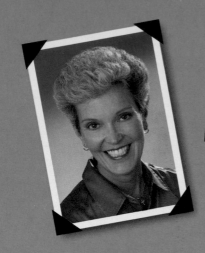

MATURE AND MARVELOUS

Nature produces beauty in youth.
Time reveals works of art.

Age is a beautiful thing. The onset of wisdom, a greater understanding of what's important and what isn't, and the ability to say "no" without guilt, are just a few of the perks that come with growing older. Time changes us inside and out, and anyone over the age of forty can attest to that. As mature women we need to realize and accept the fact that we have a different body to dress than we had twenty years ago.

It seems about the time we have the fashion puzzle all put together, gravity rearranges the pieces, and we simply must re-shuffle. Developing an attractive, age-defying wardrobe begins with stepping out of your comfort zone into the realm of *sophisticated style*. Any woman can do this, but few are willing to take the risk.

Last month, while attending a party, I had the pleasure of meeting a classy, southern lady who was seventy-two years young. Dorothy, a stunning woman with a lot of spunk, wore soft, black leather pants and matching boots with a silk printed blouse. She finished off the ensemble with gold jewelry and a smile as big as Texas. Dorothy's flattering hairstyle, touch of makeup, and tastefully put-together outfit, had most people guessing her age at fifty. Free from the need for approval, she took a risk that resulted in a look that was both vibrant and approachable.

Update and Accentuate

Start by investing in basics. Most of us in our prime have come to a point where we don't need or want as much clothing and accessories as we once did. Contentment that comes with age through buying fewer things and better quality is a smart formula for *any* wardrobe, particularly when you are dealing with the physical challenges

Smooth fabrics make skin look smoother; wrinkled fabrics draw attention to wrinkles.

that come with a time-honored body. Higher quality means a better fit and built-in structure and shape.

Get the fit right. A smartly tailored jacket or figure-flattering dress can take years off a *Shop with someone who is ten years younger and has good taste. They know the trends and will encourage you to step out of your comfort zone.* body. Frumpiness is a tell-tale sign of an older woman. Clothes that bag and sag or fold in places where they shouldn't distract rather than camouflage. Avoid droopy shoulder lines, wrinkles under the waistband, pleats that pull open when standing straight, and slacks where the crotch is either too snug or headed south. If you don't do alterations, find a professional who does.

Rediscover shoulder pads. Place them just beyond your shoulder seam so they add width and conceal a sloping shoulder line. Broadening the upper body with moderate shoulder pads will make the waist and hip area appear smaller.

Choose designs that drape for your shape. Garments that hang straight from the fullest part of your body, tummy, buttocks, or thighs, will be most flattering. Pay attention to detail. Avoid pleats that balloon out and darts that define roundness at the waist and hips. Experiment with longer, duster-style coats and vests to give a lean line and add drama to your look. Hip-length jackets with slight shaping will cover figure flaws and have you looking fabulous.

Embrace color. Lighter, brighter colors will not only reflect softer light on your face, they will also make you feel young and vibrant! Black can be attractive on some, but generally speaking, the older we get the more difficult it is to wear dark colors next to our face without appearing washed out. If you own a black or charcoal jacket or sweater, accent it with a brighter color such as melon or aqua blue in a scarf or collared blouse; collars are the most flattering since they frame the face. A hint of this same color should be repeated in another area of your outfit to complete the look.

Keep styles simple and accessories stylish. Clean lines and minimal details will serve as the perfect backdrop for trendy, chic accessories. Add some fun to your wardrobe by choosing pieces that suggest a popular print, pattern, or color that the younger crowd is wearing. For example, choose a leopard print scarf with matching shoes or try a lime green handbag and jewelry. Warning: do not go overboard! One or two places are plenty to showcase your fashion forwardness.

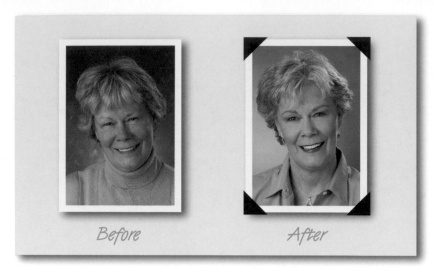

Before   *After*

Using makeup to even out Linda's skin tone softens her look as the pink blouse brightens her beautiful face. This delightful woman has a positive attitude that really shines through!

Hairstyles and Makeup

Styles change and fashion moves on, but sometimes we don't. Nowhere is that more evident than with our hair. Small adjustments such as length, part, amount of curl, bangs and side details can be tweaked to give a contemporary and fresh look. Whether you choose a cute crop, bouncy bob, or a perky pageboy, trendy tresses must be kept up. Keep regular hair appointments and remember a great cut is one that still falls into place three weeks after you've seen the hairdresser.

Carefully contemplate hair color changes by getting all the facts ahead of time and having it done professionally. Steer clear of colors that are harsh and unnatural. Having hair "foiled" with two complementary shades is a good way to refresh your color. Silver-gray hair can be ageless if your style is up-to-date. If you decide to disguise it, consider having hair highlighted with an ash blonde color to tone it down, or reverse frost it to gently minimize the gray.

Makeup should include a foundation that gives a soft glow and reflects light, not powdery or mask-like. Choose lip and cheek colors in gentle, natural rose or peach shades. Use a lip liner pencil to prevent lipstick from bleeding. Eyeshadow colors need to be soft and neutral. Avoid bright, frosted, or harsh eye makeup. Try using waterproof mascara on your top lashes *only* to prevent the raccoon effect that can occur later in the day, or with a power surge (hot flash). To make your eyes look bigger and brighter, use an eyelash curler or lengthening mascara. Keep brows well-shaped and fill in with a subtle brow color. It's best if they are one shade lighter than your hair or if your hair is white or light blonde they can be one to two shades darker. A taupe (gray-brown) powder shadow will work well for both lids *and* brows.

I strongly recommend having a cosmetic makeover done once a year by a makeup artist to help keep current on cosmetic trends and looking fresh.

Health and Happiness

> *"Middle age is when your age starts to show around your middle."*
>
> *—Bob Hope*

When you feel good, you look younger. With a proper diet and regular exercise, you can enhance your shape and posture. However, it takes *work* and *discipline*—two words when associated with our bodies we've come to detest. First, let me confess: I am a nutritional over-achiever—I love to eat. Teaching a weight loss program for the past three years has helped keep my weight in check and realize that it *is* doable. Here are some simple tips that will make the whole effort a lot easier. Choosing only one or two things to begin working on each week and build from there.

What's more important, another bite of bread or a slice of life?

SIMPLIFY YOUR DIET

- **Cut your food portions in half** and eat the rest later. This will keep your energy level at an even keel and prevent those afternoon binges.

- **Use smaller plates.** Dessert-sized plates in place of dinner plates will give the illusion of more food.

- **Eat apples and pears.** The added fiber and lower calories in these fruits has proven to curb overeating and aid weight loss by thirty percent.

- **Lower fat intake.** Try switching dairy products to skim or "light" variations, and choose low-fat breads and starches.

- **Replace soda pop with water.** Whether it's regular or diet pop, the benefits of water far outweigh the carbonated options.

- **Wear a snug belt when you eat**. This will serve as a gentle reminder of when you are full.

- **Stop eating when full.** When you've reached your capacity, push the plate out of reach. Or, put your eating utensil handles discreetly into the food to discourage you from continuing to eat.

- **Order a "To Go" box with your meal.** When eating out, before taking the first bite, place half the meal into the box. It will make an easy lunch later in the week.

- **Consume calcium.** Studies have shown that people who have diets rich in (low fat) dairy lose up to seventy percent more weight.

- **ALWAYS share your dessert.** Enjoy!

I don't live to exercise;
I exercise to live.

Exercise: a guilt-ridden word that causes people to run away! Most of us know physical fitness "does a body good," but research has also shown exercise strengthens a person mentally and emotionally as well. Staying active on a regular basis will increase energy, decrease depression, and sharpen your senses. The problem is that many of us lack the time and the energy to get started in the first place. The answer is to find a physical activity that is enjoyable and convenient to do. Then make it a priority in our daily routine.

My mother has been line dancing for the past ten years and loves it. She has maintained a healthy weight and feels great. The social interaction with friends makes it fulfilling, and the fact that she is good at it makes it fun. I accompanied her once and became humbly aware of how uncoordinated I was and how mentally sharp Mom and the rest of the group were. When they dosey-doed, I dosey-didn't, and what was supposed to be the "electric slide" landed me on my backside. I think I'll stick with my rollerblading; it's safer.

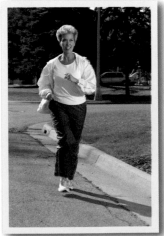

Faye is the model of living healthy. Her preferred sport is running 3-4 miles a day, 6 days a week. When she started she could barely go one block. To safely progress she made it her goal to go "a little more, never less" for the last 26 years–what an inspiration!

Dancing, bowling, rollerskating, and walking are just a few examples of activities we can choose from to keep us moving merrily along. Another good option is to try some moderate strength training. You can use two to five pound dumbbells or go to the kitchen and pull out some canned goods and baking supplies—they make excellent weights. A twenty-nine ounce can of peaches is about the equivalent of a two pound weight, or try a four or five pound bag of sugar. Using slow, controlled repetitions (eight to twelve) two to three times a week, has proven to change body composition and raise metabolism. The medical benefits include protecting bone mass and density and slowing down the effects of osteoporosis.

Morning exercisers have the most success in remaining consistent.

There are some wonderful healthy weight loss programs and fitness groups you can join to aid you in these endeavors. I have been a member of the First Place Healthy Living program for four years and have maintained my weight-loss since reaching my goal six months after joining. Information can be found at: www.firstplace.org on the internet. Another wonderful group is "Body and Soul," they provide classes and videos with aerobic exercise and strength training set to inspirational music (see www. bodyandsoul. org). For an alternative to yoga check out Praise Moves DVD and website: www.praisemoves.com. Also you can keep fit and strengthen your body at "Curves" Women's Workout Centers. They are nationwide and a great place to exercise.

Conceal or reveal?

Giving up on fashion, clothing, or style because one isn't *dazzling* anymore is a sad mistake. Many women spend the latter part of their lives wearing long sleeves, ankle length skirts, and high collars to hide their changing bodies. As one witty sixty-year-old woman told me, "Honey, some days you just have to choose between turkey-neck or turtle-neck." The mature woman can look dignified without hiding behind frumpy suits and dowdy dresses. Clothes should not distract from the real you.

Is the skin on your legs less firm than it once was? Are there so many spider veins that it resembles an accurately scaled road map of Wisconsin? Vanity tells us to cover them up so no one knows or can see. Wisdom tells us to select a tasteful pair of shorts and enjoy the breeze.

Know your age and your station. Don't try to imitate teenagers but do make an effort to keep up with the times. Dorothy reminded me that we need to modify our look as the years go by and be concerned with "the total presentation of the person" and not just the outer shell. Mark Twain put it well when he said, "Age is an issue of mind over matter; if you don't mind, it doesn't matter."

■ Living in the Moment

What is your life's purpose? If you are like me, the answer has changed over the years. When I was young, I had it all figured out: 1) graduate, 2) choose a fulfilling career, 3) get married, 4) have children, etc, etc. But with time, however, those concrete ideas that were once so black and white are now "gray" along with my hair color.

As life changes, so does our perspective. The second half of life does not mean that we move into a vacation state of mind. In Colossians 1:10 we are told to live a life, "worthy of the Lord." This verse gives us instructions on how to do just that, "…please Him in every way; bearing fruit in every good work, growing in the knowledge of God."

Please Him in every way. One way to please God is through praise. He loves to hear our praise whether in song, Scripture, or exclamation. Psalm 105:2 says, *"Sing to Him, sing praise to Him; tell of His wonderful acts."* While my singing leaves a lot to be desired, telling of His marvelous deeds, reading and quoting Bible verses, or shouting a heartfelt, "Wow!" at the amazing world He's created are all wonderful ways to praise Him.

Another way we can please God is by encouraging people with our words and actions. Be a "day-maker" for others. Look for opportunities to do "random acts of kindness," such as writing a note to the person whose smile brightened your day, kneeling down and listening to a young child face-to-face, or spontaneously filling in when a church volunteer has forgotten to show up. These works not only bring joy to those they touch, but to the giver as well. Doing things in secret is even more fun. Subtle ways to bless others might include leaving a prepared meal at a new mom's door, raking the neighbor's leaves, telling someone's boss he did a good job—the list can go on and on.

Share with God's people who are in need. Practice hospitality. (Romans 12:13)

Bear fruit in every good work. Look for the "divine appointments" God places in your day. When unexpected delays wreak havoc with your schedule, how do you react? Do you bless or stress others? When the line at the grocery store is at a standstill as the young clerk tries to change the receipt tape, use this golden opportunity to lighten her load. Turn to the person behind you, smile and start a conversation, tell a joke, or give a compliment. Before daily detours come, ask God to open your eyes to where He is working and be willing to adjust and adapt to serve Him with gladness.

For we are God's workmanship, created in Christ Jesus to do good works, which God prepared in advance for us to do. (Ephesians 2:10)

Grow in the knowledge of God. Spiritual growth is an ongoing process cultivated by prayer and meditating on God's Word. Attending a Bible study is a good way to stay sharp, but teaching a Bible study is even better. Memorize one verse a week and work it into your daily routine. Say it while you brush your teeth in the morning and again at night to help it become ingrained in your brain. You will be surprised how it can come into play throughout the day and be used to bless you and others.

Ultimately, choosing to *share* your knowledge by mentoring a younger woman is a special gift that can help her *"Live a life worthy of the Lord."* Titus 2:4 exhorts us to *"train the younger women."* This training involves sharing our life experiences and guiding others through God's Word. The opportunity to experience God's presence and power in our lives blesses both the mentor and the "mentee."

Being strengthened with all power according to His glorious might so that you may have great endurance and patience, and joyfully giving thanks to the Father, who has qualified you to share in the inheritance of the saints in the kingdom of light. (Colossians 1:11, 12)

7 SIMPLE STEPS

1. Have your clothes fitted, or re-fitted, to your body.

2. Step out of your comfort zone and buy a new trendy accessory.

3. Use color in your tops, scarves, and accessories to "frame" your face.

4. Adjust your hair color and style to flatter your features and update your look.

5. Have an *honest* friend evaluate your makeup application, then adjust accordingly.

6. *Plan* to exercise five times a week by making "dates" on your calendar.

7. Pray and look for "divine appointments."

Additional resources:
Fabulous after 50 by Shirley Mitchell
Holiness: The Heart God Purifies by Nancy Leigh DeMoss
Women of Faith Conferences (1-888-49-FAITH)

Let the beauty
of the Lord our God
be upon us."
            Psalms 90:17 KJV

Wisdom from the Bible, along with ideas and time-tested information and tools offered from my experience, are presented here to enable you to be simply beautiful.

The Creator of all things bright and beautiful invites you to know Him in a personal, intimate relationship. Only He can make us "Simply Beautiful" on the inside.

I pray that you will find yourself on a journey of renewal and contentment as you discover the beauty God has created in you and recognize the importance of nurturing the "unfading beauty" referred to in the Bible—that which will last far beyond what this life has to offer.

He has made everything beautiful in its time. He has also set eternity in the hearts of men… (Ecclesiastes 3:11)

Simply in Jesus,

Jill

For more information please visit: www.jillswanson.com
or write: Jill Krieger Swanson, P.O. Box 6291, Rochester, MN 55903